'But I'm only a social drinker...'

A guide to coping with alcohol

Dr Robert Crawford

VIKING PACIFIC

VIKING PACIFIC

Penguin Books (NZ) Ltd, 182–190 Wairau Road, Auckland 10, New Zealand
Penguin Books Ltd, 27 Wrights Lane, London W8 5TZ, England
Penguin USA, 375 Hudson Street, New York, NY 10014, United States
Penguin Books Australia Ltd, 487 Maroondah Highway, Ringwood,
Australia 3134
Penguin Books Canada Ltd, 10 Alcorn Avenue, Toronto, Ontario,
Canada M4V 1E4
Penguin Books Ltd, Registered Offices: Harmondsworth, Middlesex, England

First published by Whitcoulls Publishers 1986

This revised and updated edition published in 1991

10 9 8 7 6 5 4 3 2 1

Designed by Richard King
Printed in Hong Kong

ISBN 0670 83901 9

CONTENTS

ACKNOWLEDGMENTS

I would like to thank Alcoholics Anonymous World Services Inc., for permission to print the Twelve Steps on page 25.

Alcoholics Anonymous World Services Inc. is the official publishing arm of Alcoholics Anonymous (AA), and requests that where its literature is quoted, it is quoted in full without editorial comment. I am writing this book as a doctor who is interested in helping people who suffer from the problems of addiction, and I have frequently referred to AA and the AA Fellowship. I have done this because AA really works for people who are in trouble with booze, and because AA meets throughout New Zealand. However, my ideas and comments are not 'officially approved conference literature', i.e., literature that represents the 'group conscience' of AA. For this the reader is referred to the many excellent pamphlets and books available from the General Service Office of AA, PO Box 6458, Wellington. If I have succeeded in pointing even a few people in this direction, I will be pleased.

Thanks also go to the Christopher Smithers Foundation for the questionnaires on pages 18, 20 and 86, and to Camelot Unlimited for the Children of Alcoholics Screening Test on page 108.

The publisher gratefully acknowledges the financial assistance of the Alcoholic Liquor Advisory Council in the publication of this book.

The views expressed are those of the author.

PREFACE

I have been privileged to work in Queen Mary Hospital, Hanmer Springs, since 1972. I have seen so many patients helped, and I have kept in touch with others who did not recover, but died. Why die from alcoholism and drug dependency when help is at hand? Usually it is because defences have kept the addicted person isolated, away from support and change. This prompted me to examine more carefully what it is that 'touches the heart' and brings about the motivation for change. Always, it is something that occurs with people — a relationship with a therapist, a fellow sufferer, a friend or relation — and something that occurs within a person's spirituality. I have seen addicts make incredible transformations in a few years. I have seen others struggle without making any.

Addiction is every bit as powerful as cancer, but the remedies are jointly arrived at between supporters/therapists and patients. In cancer, the patient surrenders to medical care and all that is required is to turn up to appointments. In addiction, the therapist and patient must work together, each influenced by his or her own personality. That is why it is so rewarding when things go well, and so heart-rending when they do not.

If this book helps encourage addicted people to feel safe enough to drop their defences and talk about what is really troubling them, then I will feel it has been worthwhile.

I wish to thank my wife Jan for her support, and for criticism of the manuscript; my two sons for preventing my becoming a total workaholic; my colleagues for helpful suggestions; Miss Patricia Dunnings and Mrs Alison Hogg for patiently typing different drafts; and my patients who have taught me so much about life and addiction.

Robert Crawford

PREFACE TO SECOND EDITION

I am glad that this book appears to have helped enough people for a second edition to be printed. I have expanded the chapters on women and addiction, and adult children of alcoholics; made additions to the text about spirituality, the inheritance of alcoholism, chemical transmission in the brain, and HIV infections (AIDS). There are two new chapters. The first is on being Maori and having a drinking problem: this reflects the experience of the Taha Maori Programme at Queen Mary Hospital, and is co-authored by its director, Monica Stockdale, whose skills, guidance and forbearance have been an inspiration to me and many others. The second new chapter is an attempt to demystify psychotherapy, and is self-explanatory. I wish to thank my family for continuing to insist I lead a balanced life; and the staff, patients and ex-patients of Queen Mary Hospital, Hanmer Springs, for continuing to believe in and, more importantly, practise the philosophies outlined in these pages, often in the face of adversity and pressure.

Robert Crawford
Hanmer Springs
1991

CHAPTER 1

Should you be reading this book?

This book is for people who drink alcohol. It is also for the families of drinkers. Everybody who drinks should know what can happen when they drink too much, too often. People living and working with drinkers should also learn about the effects of drinking too much.

There is a lot to learn about why people get into trouble with booze. It is not just a matter of drinking too much — although of course this is what happens — but of what drives somebody to do this again and again. Drinkers often hurt their families deeply. Those who love them the most get hurt the most: wives of drinkers, husbands of drinkers, children of drinkers. This book contains facts about booze and booze problems that, I hope, will help drinkers and those close to them to cope with their lives better.

Although alcohol remains by far the commonest drug of misuse and addiction in New Zealand today, many people who drink heavily — particularly the young — often smoke marijuana (pot, dope, grass, cannabis) and pop pills too. A smaller number inject drugs like morphine (homebake), which is dangerous for several reasons, including the possibility of transmitting the virus that causes AIDS. Each drug produces its own type of problem, (see Chapter 16), but the underlying principles of addiction and recovery remain the same as for alcohol. If you see your problem as mainly with drugs, you will still find this book helpful by substituting the word 'drugs' for 'alcohol' whenever it occurs. I have used the phrase 'alcohol and chemical dependency' to indicate that there is a sameness about these conditions. It is now known that most mind-changing chemicals can be substituted one for another. I have seen this happen quite often with people who decide to stop drinking alcohol, for instance, but keep on smoking dope. Before long, their dope consumption has increased and they either have problems from this, or find they are back on the booze again. It is well known that recovering alcoholics who are given sleeping pills or minor tranquillisers (e.g., Valium, Ativan, Serepax, Rohypnol, Xanax, Imovane) will experience craving and may relapse.

I have learned about the difficulties that go with drinking too much by talking with people who come as patients or visitors to Queen Mary Hospital, Hanmer Springs, New Zealand. These people may be either drinkers or members of their families, and they say things like this:

Problem-drinking men

I felt so guilty, so bad inside. But I never wanted to tell anybody.

I often promised my wife I'd stop drinking, but I never kept it up.

My wife divorced me. I didn't think it had anything to do with my drinking. But it did. I was always at the pub. No wonder she got fed up. I really miss her and the kids.

I used to get terrible memory blanks. Sometimes I would have to look in the garage in the morning to see if the car was there. To see if it was in one piece.

Problem-drinking women

I felt so sad and lonely when my husband died. A drink seemed to help. Then it got so I always had a drink. The empties were a real problem.

I used to go to my bedroom, get the sherry bottle out, and get on the telephone to my friends. I'd be there half the night phoning them, sometimes.

My daughter won't speak to me any more.

My father was an alcoholic, used to make life hard for me. The only times I was happy was when I was boozed or on pills. But since I had my daughter, I know I can't stay like that.

Wives of problem-drinking men (co-dependents)

I felt so powerless. There seemed no way to turn. I was afraid of him.

I began to realise how alcohol was ruining my life — and yet I very rarely drink. So I decided to drink too for a while. But that didn't help.

I got so depressed I wanted to kill myself.

The children and I used to walk around on tiptoe for fear of disturbing him. It didn't do much good.

He used to come home from the pub and demand sex. It felt so degrading. He'd breathe his beery breath all over me and when he was finished would fall asleep at once. I used to cry silently half the night.

I knew he drank before we got married. I thought he would change.

I thought it was just his problem. I didn't realise how I was making it easier for him to carry on drinking.

Husbands of problem-drinking women (co-dependents)

I could see what she was doing to herself, but I just couldn't get her to change.

I never knew what she'd be like when I came back from work.

Sometimes she'd be her old self, and then something would upset her and she'd fly off the handle. She was so up and down all the time.

She told me so many lies I just about went crazy.

Sometimes I'd get home from work and nothing had been done since the morning. The kids would be round at the neighbour's place. It was really sad. Then the arguments would start.

She would accuse me of preferring other women. It go so bad she was driving me away. And yet I love her.

Relatives of young problem drinkers (co-dependents)

Mother: I could sense we were drifting apart, and Bob was getting more and more like his dad. But they weren't speaking to each other.

Father: He's had everything we can give him. Why shouldn't he behave himself?

Mother: I feel Shelly got into bad company early on, and didn't care about us any more. We knew she was smoking dope and drinking. But she didn't want to talk about it. I felt shut out of her life.

Brother: Ted was always jealous of me for some reason — maybe because I was a sickly baby and Mum had to devote a lot of time to me early on. I can't understand why he doesn't want to make anything of his life, just booze all his money away.

Brother: I'd get so wild at my sister for bumming around with her crummy crowd. We all knew they were into grass, and were half cut most of the time. When she got herself tattooed my father really blew his top — so she doesn't come home any more. I think she's pregnant now.

Key words

Al-Anon: Organisation for family members of alcoholics.

Co-dependents: Members of an alcoholic's family.

Degrading: Making nasty or cheap, putting someone down.

Problem drinking: Any sort of drinking that leads to problems, e.g., family rows, work rows, health problems, memory loss, traffic convictions.

CHAPTER 2

Booze problems
What are they?
Have you got one?

There are three levels of booze problems:

- *Getting drunk:* drinking too much once or twice a year. This can cause difficulties such as making a fool of yourself, vomiting, having a hangover, or more serious problems, such as having a driving accident.
- *Hazardous drinking:* drinking too much, too often. Drinking too much for your body's health, but not having many other problems — regular heavy drinking without much strife.
- *Alcoholism:* drinking too much, too often and finding it hard to control. Many problems occur, and go on occurring in spite of good intentions that they shouldn't. A variant is *periodic alcoholism*, where binge drinking occurs in between periods of normal drinking or abstinence.

All booze contains alcohol, and alcohol is a drug. It is the amount of alcohol that you drink that is important, not which sorts of booze you drink. *It is perfectly possible to be an alcoholic and drink only beer.*

We are all taught how many aspirin tablets are the right dose for treating flu; in fact it is printed on the packet. But we are not taught how much alcohol is the right dose. Some people don't like what alcohol does to them, and prefer not to drink. That is the right dose for them — nothing. After all, we won't die if we decide not to drink! Other people like the relaxing effect of alcohol, and enjoy its taste. This is their social custom and causes no problems in their lives. This is *social drinking*.

Social drinking can gradually become *hazardous drinking* if people drink more than the *safe dose*. Just as we are advised not to take more than two aspirin tablets every four hours to treat flu, so we need to know the safe dose of alcohol. The amounts in Figure 1 are given as a guide. *Note:* some people will get serious problems on less alcohol.

Remember — this is the most that is thought to be safe in one day under normal circumstances. It is not a good idea to drink up to this limit every day for two reasons:

• If you drink an amount like this every day, it may become a habit and you may gradually increase the dose without realising it, until it is too late.
• Some people are extra sensitive to alcohol, and smaller amounts than the maximum dose can still eventually cause illness in these people.

Figure 1: Approximate daily levels at which alcohol poisons the body*

(The bottles mentioned are all 750 ml or 26 fluid ounce bottles)

Men (per day)		**Women** (per day)	
Either	3 bottles NZ beer (4% alcohol)	Either	2½ bottles NZ beer (4% alcohol)
or	2½ jugs NZ beer (4% alcohol)	or	2 jugs NZ beer (4% alcohol)
or	⅓ bottle spirits (35% alcohol)	or	¼ bottle spirits (35% alcohol)
or	⅔ bottle sherry/port (20% alcohol)	or	½ bottle sherry/port (20% alcohol)
or	1 bottle wine (11% alcohol)	or	⅔ bottle of wine (11% alcohol)

All above each contain about 80 grams of alcohol

All above each contain about 60 grams of alcohol

But remember it is not wise or safe to drink this amount every day.

*The amounts given have been rounded off to give reasonable quantities —nobody is going to measure their grog intake to the last millilitre!

A guide for *moderate drinking* is:

- Not to drink every day — have alcohol-free days.
- On most drinking occasions, not to drink more than half the maximum dose.
- On special occasions, go to the maximum dose if desired.

Remember there are times in all our lives when common sense tells us the dangers of alcohol are greater than its advantages. The correct dose then is *nothing*. Examples of such times are:

- During pregnancy for women because alcohol is a drug that is poisonous to developing brain tissue in babies.
- When operating complicated machinery like piloting an aeroplane. Would you want to travel with a pilot who had been drinking?
- When told not to by a doctor for health reasons. You'd be surprised how many people seem to find this impossible!
- When driving a motor car. There are approximately 700 deaths from road accidents in New Zealand per year, and half of these are definitely due to alcohol, i.e., 350 deaths per year! This is the most common cause of young people dying in our country — and it is preventable.

Alcohol is a drug, classified as a sedative (i.e., a sleep-making drug). It has been self-prescribed since it was discovered. However, if it were discovered today for the first time, it would be a controlled drug, just like other sedatives and tranquillisers. Like any other drug in this class, the more you take, the more you need to cause its mind-changing effect. This is called *tolerance*. Somebody who can 'hold his liquor well' has a high tolerance, that is, can drink a lot before appearing drunk. Some people are born this way, but most people are not — instead, they get that way through drinking a lot. This is like a jogger getting into training. Since drinkers drink for the effect, particularly if they are heavier drinkers, they gradually have to drink more to get that effect. Unfortunately there is no tolerance to the poisoning effects of alcohol on the body, because tolerance is only for the mental effects. So heavy drinkers can poison their bodies and their brains without ever appearing drunk. The only safe way is to know the dose associated with damage, and also to apply common sense to alcohol drug taking, as you do to aspirin or blood-pressure drugs.

Recently some medical evidence has been presented which claims that small amounts of alcohol daily prevent heart attacks. The amount is about 30 grams daily. This is the amount contained in:

> 3 single hotel nips of spirits (10 grams per single nip)
> 3 hotel-sized glasses of sherry (i.e., 150 ml sherry)
> One 750 ml bottle of beer
> ¾ litre jug of beer (i.e., 750 ml beer)
> ⅓ bottle of wine (i.e., 270 ml wine)

Most doctors now think the original scientific work was faulty, and it is most unwise to rely on this idea. Not unnaturally, the greatest support for this theory comes from the booze industry itself, which is trying to promote itself as the bringer of health and happiness. It would like to forget about the vast amounts of harm done by booze.

Now let us look at the three types of booze problems — getting drunk, hazardous drinking and alcoholism. Do you have an alcohol problem?

Getting drunk

In New Zealand today, most people drink grog. Many get merry on it. This seems to be the expected thing to do at parties and special celebrations, and most of us who drink have had 'a few too many' at some time or other, and have experienced drunkenness. When we are drunk we often feel pretty good, but to an outside eye we look rather stupid, and often we do stupid things. This has been called the *illusion of performance* — but only the drunken person is fooled! Problems that people — especially young people — can have from drunkenness are:

- vomiting, hangover
- getting into fights
- losing boyfriends or girlfriends because they don't like your behaviour
- crashing cars

• out-of-character offences — burglary, damage to public property, ya-hooing.

If any of these things occur once or twice in a few years, then this may be due to drunkenness. If, however, one or more of these things keep cropping up, then a drinking problem exists.

Hazardous drinking

If you exceed the levels given in Figure 1 (page 6), this is hazardous drinking. If you drink at normal times, in normal ways, but heavily, this is also hazardous drinking. When you take alcohol regularly your brain gets used to it, so you don't get so drunk. But other problems related to drinking will gradually appear in your body, and your life. Some of these are:

Accidents after boozing	You know this one — bruises, broken bones; unexpected expenses; sick leave.
Hangover	Headaches; can't concentrate; easily irritated and upset; changing moods.
Liver damage	Pain or dragging feeling in right side of upper part of stomach area, just below ribs. Liver enlargement — can feel a lump below ribs (ask your doctor to examine you for this). Blood tests may show liver damage.
Skin changes	Red parts on palms of hands — typically red blotches at the base of the thumb and the opposite inner margin of the palm. 'Spiders': red spots on upper chest, 1 mm in diameter, with little veins coming out of them, so they look a bit like a spider with its legs. (You will need a mirror.) Red veins on face appear, with coarsening of the skin. All these skin changes are signs of liver disease.
Damage to blood-forming system	Blood tests show changes (ask doctor). Get colds and flu and infections more easily. Cuts and surgery take longer to heal.
Overweight, flabby muscles	Look in the mirror again — pot belly is a good example. Alcohol damages muscles.
High blood pressure	Headache, stroke. Often no sign but easily detected by any doctor/nurse.

Out of breath easily	'I can't run like I used to.' Alcohol damages heart muscles, cigarette smoke damages lungs — both together are therefore bad news.
Bronchitis and chest trouble	Many people who drink heavily also smoke heavily. Smoking and alcohol make lung cancer even more likely than smoking alone. Green spit. Cough up blood (always serious).
Impotence	A man can't get an erection, or only sometimes, or it is not sustained. Sex no longer enjoyable, may not bother. Fear of being impotent makes impotence more likely. May be unfaithful, as' wife not interested.
Loss of sex drive (in women)	May become passive or use sex as a weapon.
Depression, suicidal thoughts	Feelings of guilt and sadness. Poor sleeping pattern. Suicide attempts. Feeling that life is not worth the struggle.
Peripheral neuritis	Pins and needles in hands and feet. Feel unsteady, trip up easily. Weak muscles. Don't feel pain in fingers — cigarette burns may not be noticed at once. Pain in leg and arm muscles. Night cramps (this is a late sign).
Fear of heights	Gradually comes on. Avoid jobs up a ladder.
Blackouts	Temporary loss of memory while drinking —may be for short periods of a few minutes, or sometimes hours or even occasionally for days. A great puzzle for family members, who may think the drinker is lying. A frightening experience for the drinker at first — but usually tells nobody.
Brain damage	Forget things easily. Harder to learn new things, harder to concentrate, reading is harder. Suffer from mood swings, lose temper more easily. Upset by tension and stress, give up easily.

Alcoholism

When problems occur because of drink, and you try to cut down and control your drinking but can't seem to manage it so the problems keep coming back, this is *addiction*. It is like cigarette smoking. There, the body is used to having nicotine from cigarettes. If a smoker does not smoke for a while, his body sends signals that it is time he had another one. So he does! He doesn't need lots of reasons. It is just time for another one. The same sort of thing applies to alcohol addiction. But people tend to know that it is not always the right thing to do, to drink when they want one, so they try not to, even when they feel like it. An example of this is drinking in the morning. Most people know this is not normal drinking, and so don't do it. Even if you feel like it, but don't do it, this is a sign of alcoholism.

Alcoholism is a disease, in the sense that it follows a typical pattern, and also people get it and never want it, just like sugar diabetes or tuberculosis or cancer.

Signs of alcoholism include any of the things listed under *Hazardous drinking* (page 5), plus withdrawal symptoms, guilt and shame because of drinking and related behaviour, and social problems — arguments, selfishness, broken promises and so on.

Withdrawal symptoms

It isn't necessary to have them all! They start few and mild and progress as the disease progresses. Withdrawal symptoms include:

- Feeling uncomfortable after a session and knowing a 'hair of the dog' will make it better. This is the beginning of compulsion or craving, the overwhelming desire to have a drink.
- Shaking of hands. May be very slight, unnoticeable to others, or may be very obvious.
- 'Inner shakes'. Stomach churnings.
- 'Dry horrors'. Vomiting but little or nothing comes up.
- Sweats. Awake at night sweating all over.
- Hangover. Sometimes hangovers are not experienced for several years of heavy drinking, but only appear for the first time later on.
- Irritable, easily upset, argue at work and at home, mood changes.

Guilt and shame

People who have alcoholism usually know it inside themselves, but feel very guilty, and don't want to talk about it. Maori and Polynesian people often feel very ashamed. All this means is that people try to put off recognising it for as long as they can. Getting better often begins when the alcoholic realises that other people have done the same sorts of things, under the influence of alcoholism. Guilt and shame go with loss of control over drinking. You don't have to have loss of control every time you drink. Indeed, all alcoholics I have known have had control some of the time. The problem is that when they drink they do not know if this will be one of the times they are in control, or not.

Sometimes people drink quite normally except that every now and then they have a binge or a bender. Their families know this — and fear it. This is *periodic alcoholism*.

> I used to play the trumpet in a band. We'd go away to dances. About twice a year. I'd suddenly decide to keep on drinking. I wouldn't go home for several days. My wife would go frantic trying to find me. Sometimes I'd have blackouts at the same time. Later on neither of us would know where I'd been, until the bills started coming in. It was frightening. But it hasn't stopped me doing it.

Social problems

Arguments, selfishness, broken promises and the like occur a long time before most physical health problems or withdrawal symptoms. The earlier you can recognise your problem by these signs, the easier treatment will be. In this respect alcoholism is just like any other illness. In cancer, small and early growths are often cured. If you wait until it has spread throughout the body, cure is less likely.

Consult the list of examples of behaviour given below. Do any of these apply to you?

- *If you are a married woman with an alcohol problem, have you done any of the following?*

Had arguments with your husband about drinking?
Had frosty silences when your drinking is mentioned?

Carefully hidden the amount you drink?
Topped up spirit bottles with water so level is the same?
Had problems getting rid of the empties?
Had difficulties with sex life?
Said 'My husband doesn't understand me'?
Felt guilty or ashamed of your need to drink?
Found your children play up, or are too good for their own
     health, e.g., eldest daughter acts like Mum to rest of
     family?
Noticed your children do less well at school?
Felt life is too much for you?
Felt your husband is becoming more distant?
Been sexually unfaithful and felt bad?
Felt lonely and depressed, cried for no reason?
Lost your temper too easily?
Felt you are letting your family down?
Had quarrels with your mother or mother-in-law?
Broken promises to reduce and control your drinking?

• *If you are a married man with an alcohol problem, have you
   done any of the following?*

Spent less time at home?
Kept extra pay for booze money?
Cut back on housekeeping money? Got behind on bills?
Let your wife take over running and organisation of home?
Had arguments over drinking?
Hidden how much you drink?
Had problems getting rid of the empties?
Felt guilty or ashamed about treating the family this way?
Pretended there is no problem?
Broken promises to control or reduce your drinking?
Told your wife she nags you and doesn't understand you?
     Told her 'You're just like your mother!'?
Had fights with teenage sons?
Treated your children badly?
Noticed your children doing worse at school?
Not wanted to know how your children were doing at school?
Had warnings at work but not told your wife?
Lost jobs because of drinking, or left just before getting the
     sack?

Felt lonely and sad?

Spent spare time with drinking cobbers rather than with your family?

Fallen asleep in front of the TV early in the evening, night after night?

• *If you are young and single with a drinking problem, have you done any of the following?*

Spent so much on booze that you have very little to show for your money?

Crashed cars?

Been picked up for drunk driving?

Had arguments with parents and teachers about drinking?

Preferred the company of older mates when you were a teenager?

Gone on weekend parties as often as you could?

Been very rebellious as a youth?

Felt isolated and misunderstood? Hated the world?

Not been truthful about the amount you drink?

Usually tried not to leave a party until the supplies are finished?

Committed petty crimes?

Hurt the feelings of girlfriends or boyfriends?

Lost girlfriends or boyfriends because of drinking?

Drifted in and out of relationships with the opposite sex?

Been sexually unfaithful?

Found you can't remember what happened the night before?

Had homosexual encounters while drunk although not basically homosexual?

When you are wondering if you are an alcoholic, you should look at the way alcohol has affected you. The above feelings and situations have been experienced by people with drinking problems, and if some of them are familiar to you (there is no need to have experienced them all), you need to think carefully about your attitude to alcohol. Remember all the time that nobody sets out to become an alcoholic. It just happens that way, and that is why it is a disease.

Things you can do

1 Take a pencil and paper (or just think about it if you can't write easily), and make a list of the ways alcohol has caused problems in different parts of your life:

- in your family life as a youth, i.e., did your parents' or guardians' drinking worry or affect you? When did you start drinking yourself?
- in your family life as an adult.
- with money matters.
- with friends and social life.
- with your body's health.
- with legal matters.
- with doing things under the influence of alcohol you wouldn't have if you had been sober, e.g., stealing, telling lies, bending the truth, getting aggressive, being unfaithful.

Decide how serious each problem is. Remember social drinkers have *no* booze problems. Is it time to take action because of the seriousness of the situation?

2 Fill in the following questionnaires, and draw your own conclusions.

Self-administered Canterbury Alcoholism Screening Test (SCAST)

		Tick	
		YES	NO
Q 1	Have you been admitted to hospital more than once because of accidents? (By accidents, I mean all types)	☐	☐
Q 2	Have any close family members such as a parent, brother, spouse, or sister, had drinking problems?	☐	☐
	Thinking over the *last three months*:		
Q 3	Do you drink before lunch fairly often?	☐	☐
Q 4	After the first glass or two of alcohol do you ever feel a craving for more?	☐	☐

Q 5   Do you find you are thinking a lot about alcohol?   ☐   ☐

Q 6   Do you sometimes drink alcohol against your doctor's advice?   ☐   ☐

Q 7   When you drink a lot of alcohol, do you tend to eat less?   ☐   ☐

Q 8   In the morning do you sometimes feel that you might be sick (vomit)?   ☐   ☐

Q 9   Have you found that your hands have been trembling a lot?   ☐   ☐

Q 10   Have you ever used alcohol to get rid of trembling or the feeling that you might be sick?   ☐   ☐

Q 11   Have you ever been criticised at work because of your drinking?   ☐   ☐

Q 12   Do you prefer to drink alone?   ☐   ☐

Q 13   Do you think you're in worse shape because of your drinking?   ☐   ☐

Q 14   Do you ever have a guilty conscience about drinking?   ☐   ☐

Q 15   In order to cut down your drinking, have you ever felt it necessary to limit it to certain occasions or to certain times of the day?   ☐   ☐

Q 16   Do you feel you should drink less?   ☐   ☐

Q 17   Do you think that without alcohol you would have fewer problems?   ☐   ☐

Q 18   When you're upset do you drink alcohol to calm down?   ☐   ☐

Q 19   Are there times when you'd like to stop drinking?   ☐   ☐

Q 20   Would you get along better with your spouse/partner/the people you're closest to if you didn't drink?   ☐   ☐

Q 21   Have you ever deliberately tried to do without any alcohol at all?   ☐   ☐

Q 22   Have you often been told that your breath smells of alcohol?   ☐   ☐

Q 24   Write in Column 1 below the number of each type of alcohol you would normally drink *in a week* (ignore the other figures while you do this — they are for scoring the test. It looks very complicated, but it isn't really. Just follow your nose and don't panic!) Ignore Column 2 for the moment, until you get to 'Scoring' below.

	Column 1 Number		Column 2
Beer			
Glass/can		× 1 =	
Large can		× 2 =	
Handle		× 2 =	
Bottle		× 4 =	
Jug		× 6 =	
Flagon		× 8 =	
Spirits/Liqueurs			
Nip		× 1 =	
Small bottle		×16 =	
Large bottle		×20 =	
Wine			
Glass		× 1 =	
Bottle (750 ml)		× 8 =	
3-litre cask		×32 =	
Sherry			
Glass		× 1 =	
Bottle (750 ml)		×14 =	
Flagon (1.25 litres)		×22 =	
Cocktails			
Glass		× 2 =	

Box B: See

B   scoring
                        below

Box C

C

Scoring

1 Write in the number of YES's for Questions 1–22 here:

Box A

2 Multiply the number you wrote in Column 1 with the number indicated, and write this in Column 2.

3   Add all the numbers in Column 2 and write them in Box B.
4   If the number in B equals 36 or more for males, or 16 or more for
    females, write 1 in Box C, otherwise write 0.
5   Add A and C together and write Total in Box D here:

Box D   [   ]

RESULT: 0–2 — score normal limits.
            3 and more: alcohol problems severe enough for a full
            clinical assessment.

Note: This test is a screening test, designed for people admitted to
general hospitals for any condition. It was developed because
between 5 and 10 per cent of all such admissions to New Zealand
general hospitals are the result of alcohol-caused illness. It was hoped
it would be quick and efficient at helping to identify the people who
have alcohol problems. It was not intended to be fully diagnostic. Of
course it will only give an honest answer if it has been fed honest
information . . . You could check your answers by giving it to one of
the people mentioned in Question 20, and asking them to fill it in as
if they were you.

Alternatively, turn to Chapter 12, page 86, to the 'Significant
Other Questionnaire', and ask your 'significant other' to complete it
for you, i.e., girlfriend, boyfriend, spouse, family member, close
friend. If you don't like the answer you get, don't blame the tests.
They are not wrong. Instead, remind yourself alcoholism is a disease,
and re-read the section on 'Alcohlism' on page 10.

Acknowledgment
I would like to thank Mr G. A. Elvy and Dr J. E. Wells of the Alcohol Research Com-
mittee of the Canterbury Hospital Board's Working Party on Alcohol and Drug Dependence, PO Box 1876, Christchurch, for permission to use the Canterbury Alcoholism
Screening Test, and to modify the scoring slightly for publication here.

Symptoms of alcoholism

Test yourself by answering the following questions as honestly as
you can:

Physical symptoms	YES	NO
Do you crave a drink at a definite time daily?	____	____
Do you feel under tension much of the time while not drinking?	____	____
Does drinking cause you to have difficulty in eating or sleeping?	____	____
Do you at times have the shakes, extreme nervousness or dry heaves?	____	____

Do you need a drink the next morning?	_____	_____
Have you found it difficult to get work?	_____	_____
Do you lose time from work due to drinking?	_____	_____
Has your doctor ever treated you because of drinking?	_____	_____
Have you ever had alcohol convulsions, or delirium tremens?	_____	_____

Mental symptoms	YES	NO
Have you ever had a blackout (loss of memory) as a result of drinking?	_____	_____
Do you drink to build up your self-confidence?	_____	_____
Do you drink to escape from worries or troubles?	_____	_____
Have you ever felt remorse after drinking?	_____	_____
Are you at times possessed by unreasonable fears?	_____	_____
Do you have feelings of guilt or inferiority?	_____	_____
Are you very sensitive to other people's opinions, especially if they are related to your personal life?	_____	_____
Do you drink because you are shy with other people?	_____	_____
Do you at times have feelings that people are watching you, following you or talking about you?	_____	_____
Would you rather drink alone?	_____	_____

Behavioural symptoms	YES	NO
Have you become short-tempered, irritable, opinionated?	_____	_____
Is drinking making your home life unhappy?	_____	_____
Does drinking make you careless of your family's welfare?	_____	_____
Are you inclined to evade responsibility?	_____	_____
Has your ambition decreased since drinking?	_____	_____
Has your efficiency decreased since drinking?	_____	_____
Is drinking jeopardising your job or business?	_____	_____
Have you ever been in financial difficulties because of drinking?	_____	_____
Do you turn to lower companions or an inferior environment when drinking?	_____	_____
Is drinking affecting your reputation?	_____	_____

Spiritual symptoms	YES	NO
Do you lie about your drinking?	_____	_____
Are you lying increasingly as a matter of course?	_____	_____
Have you lost interest, affection or love for other people?	_____	_____
Have you become more self-centred and selfish?	_____	_____
Do you blame others for the unhappy situation in which you find yourself?	_____	_____
Do you hold bitter resentment toward certain people, and do you continue to harbour these resentments?	_____	_____
Are you still convinced that you can run your own life without help or advice?	_____	_____
Have you lost faith?	_____	_____
Have you lost your self-respect?	_____	_____

Scoring
The more 'Yes' answers, the more of a problem you have.

Stages of alcoholism

Alcoholism progresses through identifiable phases. Each phase has its characteristics. Many heavy or frequent drinkers, who are potential alcoholics, go through the initial phase without realising that their drinking is becoming abnormal. Loss of control is the hallmark of alcoholism. As illness progresses, an increasing proportion of the drinking is uncontrolled.

Directions: Place a ring around each symptom you have. This will help you picture which stage you have got to.

Beginning phase
1 Drink a lot without getting drunk.
2 Lose temper easily — pick fights.
3 Think about booze and look forward to drinking.
4 Turn automatically to have a drink when bad news received.
5 Gaps in memory ('blackouts')
6 Feel guilty inside — tell nobody.
7 Drink secretly.
8 Say you drink less than you do if anybody asks.

Early
1 When start drinking, can't stop sometimes.
2 Have a drink when don't mean to sometimes.

3 Feel guilty — talk about it sometimes.
4 Feel remorse — say you are sorry to wife/husband/girlfriend.
5 Strained relationships.
6 Make excuses for drinking. Bad behaviour.
7 Anti-social behaviour.
8 Behave like a 'big shot'.
9 Inside, feel ashamed. Don't tell anybody.
10 Attempts to give up/cut down.

Middle
1 Early morning drinking.
2 Supreme efforts to control but fail.
3 Loss of other interests.
4 Family and friends give up hope of change.
5 Physical signs, e.g., liver problems, veins on face.
6 Consult doctor about health problems owing to booze.
7 Move to new place so things will be better (geographical escapes).
8 Unreasonable resentments.
9 Withdrawal symptoms.
10 Gaps in memory ('blackouts') increase.

Late
1 Physical health problems.
2 Moral problems: tell lies, cheat, burglary, adultery, unfaithfulness.
3 Daytime drunkenness.
4 Work and money troubles.
5 Thinking is befuddled.
6 Lose all power to stop drinking unless a crisis occurs.
7 Prolonged bouts of drinking.
8 Loss of tolerance for alcohol — get drunk on less; often drunk before feel 'high'.
9 Obvious brain damage.
10 DTs.
11 Convulsions (fits).
12 Feel world is against you.

Acknowledgment
I would like to thank the Christopher Smithers Foundation for permission to use this and the preceding questionnaire, with modifications.

Key words

Abstinence/Sobriety: Not drinking alcohol at all. Sometimes used in a wider sense to mean not taking any mood-changing chemicals (e.g., cannabis) at all.

Addiction: Desire for something is stronger than reason. Slave to a habit.

Alcoholism: Continuing to drink when the evidence says it is doing you no good — addiction to alcohol.

Draw your own conclusions: Decide for yourself what the evidence means.

Drug: Anything that affects body function, e.g., alcohol, aspirin, cannabis or sleeping pills.

Exceed: Take more than.

Hazardous: Dangerous.

Illusion of performance: Belief by drinker that he or she is functioning better than normal, but outsider knows this is not so.

Moderate drinking: Keeping inside safe limits outlined on page 7.

Suicidal thoughts: Thinking life is so awful that death might be better.

Withdrawals: Symptoms felt when drinker suddenly stops drinking.

CHAPTER 3

What can you do about your booze problem?

The first thing to do is to make a clear decision about what sort of booze problem you have. Re-read Chapter 2 carefully and do the questionnaires at the end. Is your booze problem getting drunk, hazardous drinking or alcoholism? Decide what you are going to do about your problem. It is best to talk this over with either a trained alcoholism counsellor or a trusted member of your local Alcoholics Anonymous (AA) group. Better still, talk to both of them.

These are the alternatives:

PROBLEM	SOLUTION
Getting drunk Drunk once in a blue moon, causing you to have crashed car or got a single drunk-in-charge with blood alcohol below 150 mg%.	You can decide to stop before you get too drunk. Also get someone else to drive you home.
Hazardous drinking Drink too much, too often but normal lifestyle.	Make decision to reduce drinking below the levels in Figure 1 (page 5). Self-honesty vital — admit to yourself when you have failed to keep control. If you can't stick to levels then you are addicted, so move to *Alcoholism* below.

Alcoholism   Stop drinking grog completely. Look at reasons for drinking. Understand need for new interests in life to replace drinking. Consider AA programme. Consider long-term personal counselling. Consider in-patient therapy (if advised). Consider need for personal growth. Read following chapters of this book. Keep on with recovery programme in years ahead.

To recover from a booze problem, it is absolutely vital to be clear about the nature of the problem. Deciding the difference between whether you are a hazardous drinker or an alcoholic is not always easy. It is hard to admit to not having control. The image of the 'alcoholic' — a dirty old tramp in the gutter with a bottle of gin — is not typical. Top company executives, busy mothers, good-looking youths — anyone who cannot control their drinking is an alcoholic.

Most alcoholics would like to be able to drink normally and like to think they can. But we know that once diagnosed as an alcoholic, return to normal drinking is not possible. It is just the same for cigarette smokers. A cigarette smoker (or nicotine addict — it is the same thing) who stops his or her 40-a-day habit, knows that to take one cigarette will start him or her off again. The only thing to do is to stop and not smoke the first one. It is exactly the same with alcohol.

Because alcohol is a mind-changing drug, the alcoholic's situation is more difficult than the smoker's. That is why, in recovery from alcoholism, it is necessary to look at different parts of our lives in detail. It is not enough to say 'I will stop drinking and everything will come right'.

It is true that you must stop completely to start recovery, even if you do not think you are alcoholic. Only if your brain is clear (which usually requires three to six weeks of not drinking), can you make a proper assessment of yourself.

A programme of recovery from alcoholism is as follows:

- Accept that what has happened is very serious (Chapter 4).
- Understand why you became alcoholic (Chapter 5).
- Learn how to live with yourself today in order to stay recovered (Chapter 6).

- Understand attitudes that make it easy to start drinking again (Chapter 7).
- Recognise the signs of being a Dry Drunk (Chapter 8).
- Wonder if you have alcoholic brain damage (Chapter 9).
- Consider the effects of alcoholism on family life and rebuild communication with your family (Chapters 12, 13, 14 and 15).
- Know about the misuse of drugs and the pointlessness of substituting them for alcohol (Chapter 16).

You will notice this programme demands that you think about yourself, your life and the effects of alcoholism on your body. It also asks you to consider the effects on your family and relationships. You are asked to learn about drugs so as to avoid substituting them for alcohol. These are big tasks that need time and effort. They also need support from others. In Appendix 3 (page 134) you will find addresses of organisations which offer counselling and support. The most famous of these is Alcoholics Anonymous (AA), which is available worldwide.

AA has a twelve-step programme of recovery, reprinted with permission below. It is a fact that the programme has helped more people than any other become enduringly sober, and reference to these twelve steps will be made throughout this book.

Twelve Steps of Alcoholics Anonymous

1 We admitted we were powerless over alcohol . . . that our lives had become unmanageable.

2 Came to believe that a Power greater than ourselves could restore us to sanity.

3 Made a decision to turn our will and our lives over to the care of God as we understood Him.

4 Made a searching and fearless moral inventory of ourselves.

5 Admitted to God, to ourselves, and to another human being the exact nature of our wrongs. (Cont'd on p.28)

Action you should take if you have an alcohol problem

Agree an alcohol problem exists.

Talk to your family — who should read Chapters 12–15.

Talk to some knowledgeable person who will be sensitive and honest with you about it.

Decide if you are a **hazardous drinker** or an **alcoholic.**

If hazardous drinker, consider what problems occur. Discuss with people concerned.

It may help to talk to a counsellor or other knowledgeable person about your life. Do you have attitudes that cause problems? (Chapters 5–6).

If alcoholic, STOP DRINKING. Consider admission to Detox Unit. Do AA programme step 1. Accept that what has happened is serious (Chapter 4).

Recognise need to stay stopped. Live 'one day at a time' (Chapter 3).

Decide what attitudes need to be changed (Chapters 5–6). Have outpatient counselling and/or inpatient treatment. Involve your family in your recovery (Chapters 12–15).

▶ Do AA programme steps 4–5 (page 25). Deal with guilt and remorse.

▶ Be alert for BUD (page 55). Talk it out – don't act it out.

▶ Decide what support systems you need so you can face reality and face feelings (Chapter 6).

▶ Avoid substituting other mind-changing drugs (Chapter 16).

If RELAPSE occurs, it is because you haven't learned to accept and to face your alcoholism and feelings. Inpatient treatment vital (Chapter 7). Go back five steps.

▶ Do AA programme steps 6–12. Happy, loving, stable way of life opens up, with increasing ability over two years to be serene (i.e., emotional sobriety). Family begin to relax and trust.

If SOBER but LIFE NO BETTER indicates DRY DRUNK (Chapter 8). Go back five steps and seek the missing ingredients.

If hazardous drinking is only problem, stop drinking for two months (give body and brain chance to recover) and resume at lower levels. (If you cannot *stop* for two months your are probably alcoholic.)

▶ ▶ No more problems.

Continue to be vigilant of drinkings levels. *Any* recurrence of problems or if drinking creeps back to hazardous levels, indicates loss of control and addiction, i.e., change diagnosis to alcoholism.

Life much better.

6 Were entirely ready to have God remove all these defects of character.

7 Humbly asked Him to remove our shortcomings.

8 Made a list of all persons we had harmed and became willing to make amends to them all.

9 Made direct amends to such people wherever possible, except when to do so would injure them or others.

10 Continued to take personal inventory and when we were wrong promptly admitted it.

11 Sought through prayer and meditation to improve our conscious contact with God as we understood Him, praying only for knowledge of His will for us, and the power to carry that out.

12 Having had a spiritual awakening as the result of these Steps, we tried to carry this message to alcoholics, and to practise these principles in all our affairs.

Things you can do

1 Consult the chart on page 26 and decide what action is required.

Key words

Alcoholics Anonymous: Worldwide and New Zealand-wide organisation for support of recovering alcoholics. Self-supporting and not allied to any health or government agency. Address is on page 134 or in the telephone book.

Decision: To make up your mind after considering the facts, and not to change it.

Dry Drunk: Behave as if drunk or hungover, but not having had anything to drink at all. Often shows as a loss of previous serenity, which is replaced by angry mood swings, return of tension and perfectionism, being over-critical of others, being childish and demanding, etc.

Immaturity: A state of being childish, childlike.

Nicotine: The addictive drug in cigarettes.

Relapse: Go back on your decision. Drink again.

CHAPTER 4
Accept that what has happened is serious

Alcoholism is a serious condition: in New Zealand people are dying and families are breaking up every day because of it.

> I wish I had taken treatment years ago. If I'd known then what I know now, my wife and I would still be together.

> If only I had been more serious during my first admission (to hospital). I thought it was a pushover, keeping off the grog. I remember promising you I wouldn't drink, Doc.
> Do you remember what I said?
> Yes, I do. You said, Don't promise any more, just say, 'I won't drink today', but I was so sure then. I suppose I got complacent.

From the bottom right-hand corner of the front page of the newspaper:

'A man died when his car left the road at high speed and hit a power pole at 3 a.m. last night. He was the sole occupant. He was Mr J____ S____, 40, of P____ N____. He leaves a wife and two children.'

And two months later, reporting from the Coroner's Court:

'The Coroner found that Mr J____ S____, 40, of P____ N____ died from injuries sustained when his car left the road and hit a power pole. A post-mortem blood alcohol level was 250 mg%.'

The first step of the AA programme says:

Step 1 We admitted we were powerless over alcohol . . . that our lives had become unmanageable.

If you are not spiritually inclined you may have difficulty accepting some steps of the AA programme, but the first step is quite clear. All people with alcoholism must admit it, then accept it, if they want to recover. There is a difference between admitting and accepting. *Admitting* you are alcoholic is usually uncomfortable, with feelings of guilt and shame. *Accepting* you are alcoholic brings relief, and a wish to follow a plan for recovery. When we accept we are thankful to have discovered what is wrong.

How does alcohol produce addiction?

If we agree addiction is serious, the next step is to ask what is known about how it takes place. I must say straight away that nobody actually knows the full answer to this question. However, we do have some ideas which are helpful. Addiction occurs because:

- It is behaviour we unconsciously learn to do — like a trained dog.
- It is a chemical change occurring in the body as a result of drinking.
- It is a gradual process over at least two years, and usually much longer, whereby addiction becomes part of a person's way of life.

Let's look at each of these things in more detail.

It is behaviour we unconsciously learn to do like a trained dog

When my labrador Tim sees a shotgun, he gets excited. This is not because he is particularly fond of shotguns, but because he connects shotguns with shooting trips, which he enjoys. He has learned that shooting trips and shotguns are connected, through his experiences of them, not through being told that this was so. His immediate excitement at seeing a shotgun, whether it means a shooting trip or not, is known as a conditioned response. Once in place, such conditioned responses are very slow to go away. They occur easily in humans — an example is the fear we have of climbing a ladder after an unexpected fall from one.

One theory of behaviour claims it is *all* learned, that we do nothing by instinct. While most people think this is going too far, the basic message for addiction is hopeful: 'If we have learned one sort of behaviour then perhaps we can unlearn it, and behave in another way'.

In alcohol addiction, the drinker learns that boozing brings relief and pleasure in the short term, so unconsciously connects alcohol with good feelings. These short-term rewards are more valued by the drinker's unconscious mind than the longer term punishments (like hangovers, withdrawal symptoms, arguments, loss of money, health problems, etc.). This conditioned response keeps the addict at it. An example of this is:

> I was walking down the street feeling real good, Doc, when I passed this pub. I smelled the old smell, heard the chat, and thought — well, one won't hurt. I went in. Only had one, then. But you know the story, Doc, one's too many and a thousand's not enough. My urgency had gone from my recovery. I was soon back every night, even though I'd sworn to you I'd never go inside a pub again.

It seems as though very powerfully learned conditioned responses are always inclined to lurk in the mind, awaiting the right circumstances to pop up again.

> I hadn't seen my ex-wife for six months. Then we met one day when I went to collect the children. We had a flaming row. I went on a fortnight's binge the next day — and I hadn't had a drink for nearly nine months before that.

It is a chemical change occurring in the body as a result of drinking.

After it is drunk, alcohol enters every cell of the body. Just about every bodily function is affected to some degree — although the only bit we see affected is brain function. Alcohol exerts its effect partly on the outer part of each cell, and partly, it is thought, by changing chemicals that occur inside the body.

Nerve cells inside the brain work by sending minute electrical currents to each other across junctions which act like transformers in electrical circuits. Little packets of chemicals are released from one end of a junction, and cause a new electric current in the next nerve cell when they reach it. There are many different chemicals in the brain called neuro-transmitters. The pattern of neuro-transmitters we have in our brain determines how well our brain functions. Presumably we inherit our particular pattern, but it is also changed by any mind-altering drug, like alcohol or cannabis. It is thought that some people inherit a particular pattern of neuro-transmitters that makes them more likely to develop addictions.

One chemical produced in the liver when alcohol is broken down is called *acetaldehyde*. Acetaldehyde is like a paint-stripper. It is very corrosive. Because it is always produced as the body tries to get rid of alcohol, it follows that the more you drink, the more paint-stripper you will produce. Some recent research says that alcoholics produce more paint-stripper stuff than non-alcoholics, and that there is an unnatural build-up of it in their bodies. This may be inherited or may be from liver damage from alcohol itself — we don't yet know.

It is further suggested that the paint-stripper stuff (acetaldehyde) can combine with naturally occurring brain chemicals to produce substances quite like morphine. Everybody knows morphine is very addictive. It is thought that these chemicals work like morphine in the brain. It seems that once the brain has produced this special kind of morphine, it is very sensitive to it, it gets a taste for it and tends to stay 'sensitised' in this way forever afterwards.

Incidentally, it is known that hard exercise produces similar morphine-like chemicals in the brain, which may cause the 'buzz' some joggers get, and explain why they are addicted to jogging!

You can also understand how learned behaviour, the 'trained dog' response, can be reinforced by this second mechanism.

It is a gradual process whereby addiction becomes part of a person's way of life

Becoming addicted is a gradual, building-up process over a number of years. What seems to happen is that continued use of chemicals like alcohol (or cannabis, or tranquillisers) trains us to use them more, to rely on them more, instead of using other things. Who is going to 'work through their sadness' at losing a friend, if they know they can blot out all pain by drinking, even if only in the short term? Who is going to learn to overcome his or her shyness, if they know it will dissolve magically with a drink? Thus we learn not to expect to feel uncomfortable at all — take a drink (or drug) and forget. Alcohol opens the door to a lotus-eater's paradise, becoming an integral part of a person's way of life and way of looking at life. This makes addicts somewhat short-circuited in their response to the world — everything centres around alcohol in some way. It is as if addiction removes that part of a person's adult functioning that looks further ahead than the immediate future. The need for alcohol *now* is more important than any thoughts of the future.

Things you can do

1 Do you admit that what has happened is serious?
2 Make a list of ways your life is unmanageable.
3 List the ways booze has made a fool of you. Be honest —it makes a fool of nearly everyone at some stage!
4 Make a list of things that have happened to you that would not have happened if you had not been drinking.
5 How far have you got in accepting your alcoholism?
   • Are you an alcoholic?
   • Do you feel ashamed about this?
   • Do you feel angry about this?
   • Do you feel comfortable about being a *recovering* alcoholic? (Remember — most alcoholics in New Zealand are still drinking ones!)
   • Do you feel happy and relieved to know what is wrong with you?
6 Are you ready to take the first step of AA — 'We admitted we were powerless over alcohol . . . that our lives had become unmanageable'?

Key words

Admit to alcoholism: Agree to the possibility of having alcoholism — guilt and shame remain.

Accept alcoholism: Relief at knowing what is wrong; decision to follow recovery without reserve; guilt and shame vanish.

Conditioned response: A reaction that is unconsciously learned.

Inherited characteristics: Qualities we can trace back to our parents, e.g., hair and eye colour, shape of face, tolerance for alcohol, intelligence, etc. Also called genetic characteristics.

Unmanageable: Out of control.

CHAPTER 5

How did you get to be an alcoholic?

As well as the three processes described in the last chapter (unconscious learning, chemical changes, and addiction as a way of life), there is a need to understand two other contributing factors. These are the social customs of the country, and the mental make-up or personality of the addict.

The social customs of New Zealand

We need not spend long on this one. The basic idea is that the more people who drink alcohol (or take drugs), the greater will be the number who become addicts. This fact is so obvious it hardly seems necessary to state it. There were large numbers of people with alcohol problems in Victorian times, and there are large numbers now. In between these times there were not so many alcoholics, because of restrictions on the availability of booze (with short licensing hours, introduced early this century) and because there was less money around (the Depression). As soon as New Zealand got wealthier after World War II, and 'six o'clock closing' was done away with, it is a fact that the amount of alcohol drunk doubled. If we now add in the pressure on young people to drink because it is 'the thing to do', then we have a system which ensures people meet alcohol, often in large quantities.

There is, therefore, an element of chance in whether people drink alcohol. If you had been born 30 years earlier, or in a country where people don't drink much (e.g., Israel or Saudi Arabia), probably you wouldn't have become an alcoholic.

The mental make-up or personality of the addict

If it is your luck to be born into a country where a lot of alcohol is drunk, then you also need to select your parents with care! This is because some of our mental make-up is inherited; some is the result of the training we receive from our parents when quite young; and the rest is the result of how the world treats us and our reactions to it.

Everyone knows that all human beings are capable of acting childishly at times. Mature people can be thrown off guard by severe stress; less mature people are affected by less stress. Alcohol problems cause childish, selfish attitudes in varying degrees, according to the individual's mental make-up or personality.

Some people's mental make-up makes them very vulnerable to mind-changing drugs and 'magic' potions, often without their realising it. During treatment it is necessary to look for reasons in your mental make-up which might have contributed to your alcoholism. Then you need to try to change these. You can't change your personality, but you can struggle to alter mental attitudes. Often, the realisation of hidden feelings about matters that may have puzzled you is enough to bring about mental growth, and to separate you from ever-repeating past cycles.

> Until I went to psychodrama, I never realised how much I really loved my mother. I thought I hated her, and was pleased when I left home at 15. I'm 30 now and want to change my relationship with her.

> My little brother, who was hyperactive, got run over. He was two and a half and I was seven. I'd always felt responsible for his death. In later life I've taken all sorts of risks with my life, somehow feeling I didn't deserve to live. I've had so many traffic accidents, it's not funny.

> I've never been close to my eldest boy. And yet I love him. I guess he is too like his dad, who got killed when we'd been married for two years.

Sometimes people sense there is something wrong with their inner functioning, but never make progress in discovering what it is. One reason is that you can't do it alone. You must work these things through with a therapist. If you are a Dry Drunk then there are hidden feelings inside you which are part of your mental make-up. With a good therapist you can begin to see what they are, but it is a fact that you won't make progress in this area on your own, or (alas) just by reading this book. I am writing this to encourage you to work with a therapist or counsellor on such problems and also to attend a growth group. Reading Chapter 17 on Psychotherapy may also help.

Often when you act childishly it is a defence against anxiety. You feel anxious, but rather than experiencing and working through your anxiety, you substitute a defence — that is, you do something that avoids the problem without actually solving it. This is perfectly natural, but some defences just add to your problems. For example, if you turn to drink or drugs; or move from one place to another, thinking that this will solve your problems (geographical cure); or react with irrational anger and resentment, your problems will be made worse, not better. Behind the anxiety and the defence you must look for the hidden feelings that make you behave as you do.

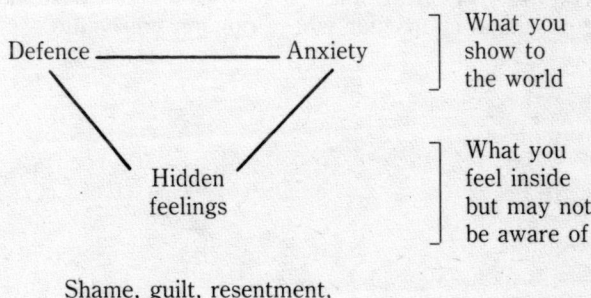

When you were born, you were full of potential. The things that happened to you on your journey since being conceived and later born, plus your inherited characteristics, have made you what you are today. You can think of all your childhood, adolescent and later experiences as the training you received for life. Often there are many things that have happened to us that have left scars on our mental make-up, just like a wound on the skin that leaves a mark forever. Just as a skin wound can be altered by plastic surgery, so can a mental scar be modified by suitable therapy. If you have plastic surgery because you want to change, you are prepared to put up with some discomfort. It is the same with personal growth therapy — you must be prepared to experience discomfort for later gains.

Things you can do

1 Make a list of situations that cause you to behave less well than you would like. Are your reactions justified, or not? For example, how do you react when you are tired; when you do not get your own way; when you are being asked to do too many things at once; when you feel under pressure; when you've been drinking; when someone is rude to you; when someone is critical of your drinking?

2 Are you in touch with why you behave poorly? If not, you need more insight. Talk it over with a trusted friend, or a professional counsellor whose opinion you value.

Key words

Anxiety: Fears about something in the future.

Dry Drunk: Behave as if drunk or hungover, but not having had anything to drink at all. Often shows as a loss of previous serenity, which is replaced by angry mood swings, return of tension and perfectionism, being over-critical of others, being childish and demanding etc.

Geographical cure: Move from one place to another, thinking the move will cure alcohol and drug problems.

Growth group: Group run by therapist aiming to promote personal understanding and help people live more happily and cope better.

Hidden feelings: Feelings that may be unconscious or of which we are only dimly aware.

Inherited characteristics: Qualities we can trace back to our parents, e.g., hair and eye colour, shape of face, tolerance for alcohol, intelligence, etc. Also called genetic characteristics.

Inner functioning: What we really feel, deep down inside, but do not usually tell anybody.

Magic potion: A wonderful drug you expect to act like magic.

Mature: Behave in an adult way; opposite of childish.

Stress: Feeling of being required to do too much, having too much on your plate.

Psychotherapy: Any attempt to relieve a person's mental distress by mental means, e.g., by talking or by thinking in new ways.

CHAPTER 6

The recovery process

Get a grip on what happened in your life and addiction, and learn how to live with yourself today

Alcoholism is a disease that can affect anybody. Kind people, rough people, clever people, dull people — anyone can get alcoholism. Because all alcoholics are guilty and ashamed, deep down inside, it is necessary to do something which clears out the past things we would rather forget but cannot. From helping alcoholics over many years, I know that the past can never be forgotten. Indeed it must not be forgotten because, 'Those who forget the past will relive it.'

Instead, we must find a way of coming to terms with painful memories. Here are some ways of doing this:

- Go through your life history with a counsellor or therapist.
- Think about your spiritual position.
- Do steps 4 and 5 of the AA programme.
- Face up to severe losses in your life.

These will now be considered in more detail.

Go through your life history with a counsellor or therapist

You will need to trust your counsellor. If you cannot, tell him or her so. Obviously it will take time to get to know him or

I am grateful to Father John Prendergast, SM, for some of the material in this chapter.

her, so immediate trust is not usually possible or the best. As you tell the counsellor about your life, try to talk about the feelings you have about things that have happened. Explore these. With a good counsellor you may be surprised at what you discover about yourself.

There is no recovery without self-honesty. Do not be surprised if your counsellor says some hard things to you — the truth about ourselves is always hard to take. Try to get your half-thoughts, half-feelings out into the open. This will make them easier to come to terms with. Keep an open mind and don't think that you have no inner feelings, because dealing with inner feelings is the key to a happy recovery. Some doctors think that some people become addicts because they never learned to express their feelings in words — they learned instead to drown them in a sea of booze. To change that you must stop the booze, clear your head, and try to learn to express yourself. You will find your counsellor will respect you more if you are honest and open, whatever bad things have happened. This respect will make it easier to learn to express your feelings. Joining a group of other recovering alcoholics will also help with this.

Think about your spiritual position

If you are an alcoholic, you know what a powerful disease alcoholism is. Under its influence you say and do things you later wish you had not. And yet, before long, having decided not to, you do them again. In varying degrees you will find yourself tense, selfish, and wrapped up in your own welfare — but often to little avail. You will feel worthless, hopeless and alone. At times like these you will wonder, 'What is this life for?' When you ask a question like this, you are asking a spiritual question.

As soon as the word 'spiritual' appears, many readers will immediately think of dull churches, or stuffy religion, or cruel nuns/brothers at school, and at once read no more. This is a mistake, because spirituality has not necessarily got anything to do with organised religion. If I look out of the window now, I can see grass, trees, some birds flying past, a cloud being pushed across the sky by the invisible wind. I can also be conscious of planet Earth in the vast caverns of space, and tonight there will be a moon and stars. I realise how small I am, and how little I know — indeed how little mankind really knows. There have been generations before me, and there will be generations after me. Nature's creatures and nature's forces will continue on, around and within me. I am a part of this vast moving universe and there is only so much I can do to influence it. More often it will be a case of flowing on with the current, doing my best to swim efficiently, and trusting in the unseen forces. I will try to be clear about my little area of responsibility, and will do my best with it. The larger area I will have to hand over to whatever I understand by the unseen forces. If I can believe in some sort of Higher Power which has my welfare at heart in some sort of way, then I will not feel so alone — I will become a part of the world around me.

For some people, this Higher Power will be nature: they will identify with the life force in humans, animals and plants. For others, it may be the power for good in a group of people (e.g., a therapy group, or an AA group, or a church group). For others, it may be some sort of religion. In New Zealand many people can reaffirm their faith in some form of Christianity: it may be necessary to update our belief system from the childish 'Old Man in the Sky' to a more adult view. For many people, other religions may be more helpful, e.g., Baha'i, or Eastern philosophies. But it is perfectly possible to have a healthy spiritual position without subscribing to any form of organised religion.

For some people, spiritual awakenings come suddenly. Bill Wilson, the founder of Alcoholics Anonymous, had one of these which is described in the book about him, *Pass It On.* (See Further Reading, page 128). For most people, spiritual awakenings are smaller events, gradually adding up to a faith as time passes and we become more mature, appreciating what a mysterious place our world is. 'We are more than our thoughts, more than our bodies.' Try to interpret steps 2 and 3 of the AA programme in your own particular way.

Step 2 Came to believe a power greater than ourselves could restore us to sanity.

Step 3 Made a decision to turn our will and our lives over to the care of [our Higher Power]* as we understood [it].*

The really important thing is to end up with a belief which answers the question 'What is this life for?', and which supplies the ability to trust enough to hand over worries and anxieties. 'Let go and let God' is one slogan which enables craving addicts to take a step backwards from the brink, and retain their sobriety. Chapter 6 of the 'Big Book' (as the book *Alcoholics Anonymous* is known) explains all of this more fully.

If you still have difficulty, some people have found help in following the advice to 'act *as if* there is a Higher Power', and find that this helps to get them over a crisis. Nobody can really define a Higher Power — it is more of a feeling of something much more powerful than ourselves.

Do steps 4 and 5 of the AA programme

Step 4 Made a searching and fearless moral inventory of ourselves.

An inventory is a list of good and bad points about yourself. A practical way is to write (or tape-record if you find writing difficult) the story of your life. Go through the various stages of your life, recording all the little incidents that stand out as important and how you felt about them then and now.

1 Early childhood years — were they happy or not? How did you get on with your parents, your brothers and sisters?

2 Primary school years — how did you get on with work/play/teachers/other pupils?

3 Secondary school years — how did you cope? Were you rebellious? Did you feel inferior? Shy? Did you prefer older company?

4 Were there any sexual problems? Have you had any homosexual encounters?

5 How did you cope with work? What jobs have you had?

6 When did you first start to drink?

7 When did you first get drunk?

*These are my words in the brackets — see page 25 for AA words.

8 What sort of friendships did you make — with men? with women? Make a list of special friends you've had.

9 Have you broken the law? How often?

10 If married — what were your dreams and how did they match up with what actually happened? How did your drinking affect your marriage? How did you treat your wife and children?

11 When you look back, when did you first begin to have a drink problem?

12 Why did you not come to treatment earlier?

13 What was your attitude to your problems a few weeks ago, compared to now?

14 What people have you hurt the most?

Having done this, read it through. See if you can recognise the pattern of your life. Try to see what you have done right, and where you have gone wrong. Try to get in touch with your ideals, your best thoughts. If you once had comfort from belief in a God (Higher Power), try to work out why you stopped believing. Often people keep drinking because they feel bitter and angry about things that have happened. Can you tell where your bitterness comes from?

It is helpful to see the following checklist of personal values. When in your life have you functioned in these ways?

Positive behaviour	*Negative behaviour*
Sharing	Selfish
Optimistic	Pessimistic
Happy	Depressed
Humility	False pride
Admitting mistakes	Perfectionism
Being yourself	Being phoney
Patience	Impatience
Feeling good about yourself	Self-pity
Forgiveness and understanding	Resentment
Tolerance	Intolerance
Being honest, facing reality	Alibis, excuses, dishonesty
Getting the job done	Putting things off
Freedom from guilt	Guilt feelings
Acceptance	Fear
Being grateful	Taking things for granted

When you do your inventory, you should try to be aware of your positive behaviour, as well as of your negative. Nobody is all negative. Recovery consists of bringing out and enjoying the positive and cutting down the negative.

Step 4 should be done thoroughly in the first few months of sobriety. But it is never really finished. You will need to come back to your inventory again and again in the months and years ahead. This is recognised in step 10 of the AA programme.

Step 10   Continued to take personal inventory, and when we were wrong, promptly admitted it.

Step 5 is necessary if we are to forgive ourselves for the pain our disease has inflicted on others:

Step 5   Admitted to God [Higher Power], to ourselves, and to another human being the exact nature of our wrongs.

The 'other human being' may be a minister, a counsellor or a friend you trust who knows about alcoholism. It is preferable to have somebody you don't know well and will not meet every day afterwards. It is vital you completely trust them, so you hold nothing back.

Face up to severe losses in your life

Some people's alcoholism is closely bound up with grief — for the loss of a loved one, by death or separation, or for the loss of a normal childhood with loving parents. There may be grief over losing jobs, possessions or status through alcoholism and there may even be grief for the loss of alcohol itself. If grief is a problem it requires treatment (see page 50: Your attitude to your inner feelings). Here are some examples of grieving:

> My wife left me because of my drinking. I came back from work one day to find the furniture was gone. There was just a bed and a few knives and forks. I didn't know where she'd gone. Took the kids too. I was so lonely. She'd often said she'd go, but I never thought she'd do it. After that, well, I just gave up. There didn't seem to be any point in getting sober. Now I know I have the choice for my own life — I'll get better because I want to. But I do feel sad about Marama.

I lost my shearing contract through booze. I felt so ashamed —
my uncle took it on and he's not half as good as me. I went on the
razzle after that. It seemed the end.

After Don was killed, I felt really bad. He drank and I'd shouted
at him just before he left in the car. I thought I was responsible
for his death somehow. I felt so guilty. I only felt better when I
had a few. Since I've been to Grief Group, I realise I wasn't
responsible for his death. He'd actually have wanted me to fix
myself up, maybe marry again.

Getting struck off the Register [of Medical Practitioners] was the
worst thing that ever happened to me. I was so angry — rope-
able. I drank twice as much after that. Sometimes I'd weep, but
I'd never let anybody see that. Now I'm coming to terms with it.
They were right to do it. I will plan to work my way back again
— sober this time.

I got quite depressed during my early sobriety. It was as if I was
mourning everything that had happened. I was glad I was sober.
But I was sad it was necessary.

Grief therapy consists of re-experiencing the emotion in a
supportive setting, properly expressing the sadness. Different
people do this in different ways, but I have seen role play,
psychodrama and joining a grief group help many people.
This may need several sessions, spread over time — or a
single session may suffice. The only rule is to be guided by the
results. If you need more, then ask for it.

Things you can do

1 Are you clear about the need to do a personal inventory
   (Step 4)?
2 What prevents you from starting?
3 Do you have somebody confidential to share it with (Step
   5)?
4 Are there deeper conflicts you are becoming aware of
   which require deeper therapy, such as:
   • Resentment
   • Grief/loss
   • Rebellion
   • Problems from immature attitudes
   • Problems in relationships, in marriage, de facto, or at work

- Influence of parents' attitudes on you now
- Adoption

If so, talk to a counsellor about them.

Key words

Addict: Person dependent on drugs or alcohol.

Ashamed: Feeling of being judged unworthy or a disgrace by others.

Counsellor: Person trained to help with difficulties experienced in life.

Craving: Urgent need for a drink or a drug.

Grief: Feeling of sorrow, great mourning for a loss of any kind.

Guilt: Feeling of having done wrong or of being bad; self-blaming.

Higher Power: The Life Force; the power for good in humans; God as we understand him/her/it.

Inner feelings: Thoughts and emotions we tend to keep to ourselves.

Inventory: Complete list of everything.

Resentment: Inner feelings of injury or affront; a sort of smouldering anger.

Selfish: Self-centred, one-sided, possessive, see only own point of view.

Spiritual: To do with our soul, our vital being.

Tense: Uptight, strained, on edge, restless, can't relax.

Therapist: Usually a paid counsellor trained to a high level.

Trust: Dependable, can be relied on, worthy and confidential.

CHAPTER 7

Attitudes that make it easy to start drinking again

Anyone who has alcoholism has got into a state of mind called 'Drinking Thinking'. Drinking Thinking describes the attitudes that an alcoholic has towards other people, himself or herself, and life in general. These attitudes control our actions and reactions. You may have had some of them before you started drinking, and drinking has intensified them, while others have developed as a result of your addiction to booze. It is as if the addiction trains you to react in certain ways, even when you are not drinking.

Your attitude to the alcohol scene

For alcoholics, drinking is a priority. Everything is organised around the need to drink. Some recovering people tell themselves that they keep going back to the pub or club 'for the company': 'I'll just go down to the club as usual after work and have a juice or lemonade.'

Who are they kidding? The whole alcohol scene is still very important to them and they are doomed to failure in their search for a happy sobriety. They will either not be able to keep up drinking just fruit juice when their mates are all getting 'nicely thank you' week after week, or they will become resentful that they cannot drink too, and build up a lot of anger inside themselves. They become a Dry Drunk — someone who is chemically sober, but not feeling comfortable about it.

Changing your attitude so that you base your life around something other than drink isn't easy, but the rewards are very great. You have formed a deep and intimate relationship with alcohol; now you have to put something else in its place for your special needs. It needn't be one thing only — many things can become important to you once you stop drinking, including family, friends, a Higher Power, work, sport and hobbies.

Gain an attitude of acceptance

The best way to start changing your attitude to alcohol as the most important thing in your life is to accept fully that you are no longer able to drink it: it is poison to you. Once you believe this fact in your heart of hearts, then you will have accepted it. There is a clear difference between admitting and accepting. Admitting is often a reluctant, grudging process:

> Yes, I suppose I'm an alcoholic, better try to stop drinking for a while . . .

Acceptance brings relief, as if a weight has been lifted from your shoulders:

> Yes, I am an alcoholic but I don't want to drink any more. I'm going to do all I can to stop drinking and look forward to a great sober future. I can see that there is no situation that drink will improve for me. I will face everything straight.

Things that help you to accept are:

- Remembering the bad things booze has done to you — it is helpful here to go to AA and share these memories with others.
- Reminding yourself that you are a worthwhile person and it's not a sin to get alcoholism.

> I was riddled with guilt — for being unfaithful to my husband, for letting my children down, for being an alcoholic, just for being me! I thought I was going crazy. As soon as I understood alcoholism was a disease, I began to make amends — like it says in Steps 8 and 9 — and I found people were really understanding. They knew I'd been a drunk but they still talked to me. When I could see that, I began to get a little self-respect back. Thank God for sobriety!

Watch out for an attitude of complacency

Acceptance needs to be continued, every day. After 18 years of sobriety, one AA member had this to say:

> I don't go to AA meetings regularly every week any more, but I go occasionally. I keep my name on the Twelfth Step* roster. I find a call out to talk to some chap in a drunk crisis reminds me I can relapse too.

This man never let himself get complacent, but it is all too easy to be like a more recent 'recovery', and think that one little drink won't hurt:

> I had been sober for six months when I met an old friend and his wife, in the street. We got talking, and he invited me in for a quick one. I knew I ought to have told him I was an alcoholic, but I suddenly felt shy, and didn't like to say. After all, what was it to do with him? But I went in and had one. Handled that all right, too. Didn't tell my wife when I got home, but she knew, I think. Soon I was back to my old tricks.

Your attitude to your inner feelings

Booze has played havoc with your feelings. It has helped you bury some of them (guilt, shame), it has numbed some of them (grief, hurt), it has allowed you to express some of them (joy, anger). Now you have to cope with your feelings all by yourself — or do you?

Anger, sadness, depression and guilt are all feelings that you will need to recognise in yourself as you go through everyday life. Then you need to deal with them in a constructive way. These feelings in particular need to be *talked through* with an understanding friend, not acted out on your long-suffering family or workmates. Remember the slogan:

Talk it out, don't act it out

Often it is best to seek professional help from a counsellor, clergyman or doctor when learning to deal with your feelings. If your feelings keep landing you in more serious problems

---

*Step 12: Having had a spiritual awakening as a result of these Steps, we tried to carry this message to alcoholics, and to practise these principles in all our affairs.

you may need deeper counselling, such as will occur in group therapy, growth groups, psychotherapy, grief counselling or psychodrama. There is no shame attached to such therapy; and it may make a big difference to your recovery.

> I never realised until I had a psychodrama session how my fear of women was bound up with my drinking.

> I got off the grog okay but I get so depressed. My doctor gave me antidepressants and they helped a bit. But I don't want to take pills all my life, so I came to Queen Mary and really had a look at myself. My therapist sent me to Grief Group, and I buried my mother again. I wasn't allowed to go to her funeral when I was a lad, you see. I've felt a lot better since then.

> Since I've been coming to therapy, I've learned how I can talk about feelings — but I don't really allow myself to feel them. That's why I think I was a Dry Drunk the last eighteen months. I never was allowed to feel them when I was small — always pleased other people — so it's quite new to me, this whole area.

Relapse can ocur very easily when people allow themselves to be overwhelmed by their feelings. If you can keep recognising and understanding your emotions, and can see beyond the immediate present, keeping up your hope for the future, then you can endure through troubles pressing you now. Remind yourself that if you avoid drinking, you keep the upper hand over your situation and feelings. Take a drink and you may find relief for a few hours, but the problems are still there, and have usually been made worse by your drinking. Serenity comes over a long period of time from learning not to be overwhelmed by short-term feelings, and to cope with them without using addictive chemicals.

Happiness and joy are emotions which we sometimes find difficult to feel and express, especially without alcohol: 'You're a funny fellow. You seem to have a happy time without booze.' That remark was made to a recovering alcoholic at a party. It demonstrates the ridiculous myth that apparently it isn't possible to have fun without being drunk or stoned. If non-addicts can have fun when boozed, without it leading to further problems, then they can consider themselves fortunate. Alcoholics can't. Therefore you need to learn how to 'let go' and have fun at the odd festive occasion, family picnics and outings, dances, AA gatherings, or just when relaxing at home with the kids — without resorting to chemicals to change your mood. Adopt a positive attitude — when you are happy, share this feeling with others by expressing it in your words, your face, your movements.

Recovery sometimes seems very serious and dull — which is why you are encouraged to find a way of expressing and developing your sense of fun in your own way. Yarning, telling jokes, trying new things for a giggle, being active and positive instead of passive and negative — it is possible, if you decide that it's worth making the effort.

Many people find it satisfying to express themselves through writing, poetry, painting or learning to dance — or any artistic effort, in fact. If you feel these creative urges welling up in you, go for it! They are all part of healthy living.

When you have succeeded, you may find you have a more mature attitude to life than a great many social drinkers. You will end up saying, 'I am pleased to be a recovering alcoholic.'

Your attitude to relationships

Life is more positive when you have good relationships with those who are near you at home or at work. You are only 50 per cent responsible for any relationship; the other person is responsible for the other half. Where relationships are difficult, e.g., you feel a workmate is on your back all the time, you may need to keep reminding yourself of this, and learn to walk away. This does not mean bottling everything up — it just means you are learning to cope with your feelings without the help of alcohol and need to take it gently. The earlier in recovery you are, the less advisable it is to lose your temper. Instead, go to your sponsor, counsellor, or trusted friend (trusted to be sensible and confidential) and let your feelings out there. That is a safe place to express them. Then you won't nurse a resentment and feel like drinking.

When somebody is upsetting you . . .
don't try to argue with them . . .
go and talk out your feelings with your counsellor/sponsor

Getting emotionally involved (falling in love; being infatuated; thinking somebody else is wonderful) is a dangerous time, particularly for alcoholics in early sobriety. You will need to be honest with yourself about your basic intentions and inner feelings. Are you just looking for someone to depend on, now that you can no longer depend on alcohol? There's nothing like falling in love to make you feel better about yourself for a while — but it won't change your basic attitude to yourself, it just makes you think about someone else at a time when you should be thinking hard about yourself and your problems. You may also rush into relationships in your eagerness to replace those that have been lost through alcoholism, but so often it will lead to the past repeating itself, in a new situation. At our hospital, the staff are always on the lookout for such situations developing, and work to stop them, because they are *always* disastrous.

> Last time I was here [at Queen Mary Hospital] I got asked to leave for pairing off. Well, it's true we did go off together, but it only lasted a few days. I woke up to what I had done — stupid really, when you were all telling me. I suppose I am stubborn. I've learned the hard way. I won't be making the same mistake again.

Emotional dependency can occur between people of opposite sexes, or the same sex, and leads to isolation from reality. I suggest you avoid new emotional entanglements for the first one or two years of sobriety.

In alcoholism you hurt the most those who love you the most — husbands, wives, children, parents. These are the people about whom you will feel the most. Your emotions will often be quite different at different times. Be prepared to have different, even opposing, feelings about one person at the same time. Don't expect everything to be cosy and wonderful, just because you are sober. You have merely joined the normal world, and must set about living with your feelings like a non-addict has to, instead of blotting them out with booze or chemicals. Make sure you get support from real friends or professional counsellors during this time. Consider joint counselling.

Anger management

Sometimes sobriety brings with it a new tendency to anger. If this happens to you obviously you have not got peace of mind. You will need to get help from a trained counsellor about how to recognise the building up of that anger, and how to defuse this. As mentioned on page 52, the key is to talk about these feelings early on to your sponsor or a trusted friend.

Your attitude to getting your own way

Alcoholics are often very sensitive people. They are particularly sensitive to criticism, and often feel they have to prove themselves by being right all the time. They don't like to feel someone else is getting the upper edge: 'If I let him have his way, he'll rub my nose in the dirt, I'll be in the gutter. No, I'll make sure he pays.'

If you are to enjoy any peace in your life, this attitude has to change. At this point you may say, 'You want me to be a doormat, do you?' or 'Am I supposed to give in to everybody else?' The answer on both counts is an emphatic 'No'. All you need to do is see the other person's point of view, the other side of the argument. It is never a sign of weakness to do this, it is being open-minded, which is a sign of strength. People who always try to get their own way but do it in a less obvious way are often called 'manipulative' people.

> My husband was always so hard to communicate with. I had the feeling he was only telling me what he wanted me to know, as if he didn't quite trust me. It absolutely exasperated me. He used to arrange things behind my back and then present them to me — too late to change. Important things, like shifting home, and little things too, like being late home and telling me fibs about where he'd been. I know he'd been at the pub and not where he said he'd been.

If you don't change your attitudes, what then?

Hanging on to your negative attitudes will often lead to a build-up of bad feelings inside yourself. This will make you want to drink. You may suppress this desire and not recognise it for what it is. However, your body will usually express it to you in what is called a BUD (Building Up to Drink). There are cer-

BUD — Building Up to Drink (or Drug or Eat)

Starting point	Initial zone	Up zone	Acute zone	Solutions
Tension headaches. Back and shoulder pains.	Mood swings bigger. May say, 'I want to leave the programme.'	Irritability obvious to patient and others. Emotional inebriation has occurred.	Loss of control (patient will drink). Incapable of reason. Incapable of recalling previous disasters. Incapable of foreseeing beyond the next drink.	(1) **Drinks again.**
Tightness in stomach. Perspiration (cold sweats).	Will say, 'I have got alcoholism beat and will provide my own solution.'	Overly concerned with minor matters, e.g., resentments, money, imagined insults.		
Breathing difficulties. Eating problems. Sleeping problems. Constipation. Palpitations.	Will miss appointments. Will stop Antabuse. Will stop other medications.			
Female: periods fluctuate.	May experience depression.	Needs to talk about feelings but won't.		OR
—	Mild tremors. Marked perspiration. BUD noticeable to others.	Looking for excuses to drink.	—	(2) May dissolve the BUD by **talking** — before reaching the acute zone.
Overexcitement. Mood changes. Expressions of boredom. Loss of interest in therapy groups. Increase in tiredness.	Patient often not aware of BUD.			
—	Keeps bottling up feelings.			
Bottles up feelings — doesn't tell anyone about feeling bad.				

tain physical and mental symptoms which signal the onset of a BUD. These are different for different people, but most people experience several of the symptoms shown on this chart.

You should know what your own particular type of BUD feels like, and be able to take action to prevent it getting worse. Talking about how you feel will (amazingly) cure a BUD. Your AA sponsor can play a valuable role here. It is vital for you to be able to tell when a BUD is coming on, and talk about it to your sponsor, counsellor, or an understanding friend. Any delay is serious — your body is telling you that you must drink and this is an emergency for the alcoholic.

Into action

In this chapter I have written about understanding and changing attitudes. If you only think and talk about change, and never make the effort needed to do it, then you are only working with your brains (intellectualising) and nothing will come of it. You have to put words into action. Often this seems like jumping in at the deep end of a pool when you are not sure of your swimming ability. You must find the courage to try new ways of behaving. Every time you handle an old situation in a new and better way, you will feel a sense of achievement, and it will be easier the next time. So — with support from your friends and your Higher Power, take courage to change the things you can, and *act* in a way you know is best.

Things you can do

1 Give up your old drinking haunts; find new places to socialise; take up new interests.
2 Make a list of the most important people and things in your life and decide that you are no longer going to let alcohol get in the way of your enjoyment of these people and things.
3 Look in the mirror and say, 'I'm a recovering alcoholic and I'm okay.' Do this every morning when you get up.
4 Go regularly to AA.
5 Keep an anger diary: note down all the times you feel irritated or angry, what makes you so, and what you do with

your anger (act it out, bottle it up or talk it through with someone).

6 List the things that make you happy. Choose one of them to do each day.

7 Each time you are happy, make a habit of telling someone else about it.

8 List the good things about your relationships with your spouse, parents, children, friends, then list the bad things. Discuss this list with your counsellor or sponsor.

9 Next time you have an argument say, 'You could be right, convince me', and see where you end up.

10 Make a list of your own BUD symptoms. Stick it up somewhere where you can see it.

11 Make a list of your AA sponsors (it is often advisable to have more than one, if possible) with their telephone numbers. Stick it up where you can see it.

Key words

Acceptance: Attitude of being comfortable and happy with diagnosis of alcoholism.

Anger: Lose temper; feel tense, aggressive; prickly, spiky attitude; often masks inner sadness.

Attitude: The way a person looks at life, e.g., a serene attitude or an angry attitude.

BUD: Short for 'Building Up to Drink (or Drugs or Eat)'. A series of events and feelings that may lead to relapse.

Complacency: Gradually forget severity of previous alcohol problems; stop attending recovery programme (e.g., stop AA, stop Antabuse, stop reading the 24-hour book); stop being grateful for sobriety and take it as a matter of course. Often followed by Dry Drunk and then relapse.

Drinking Thinking: Losing touch with sad/bad behaviour of active addiction. Cease to be humble and grateful. Return to 'only I know best' attitude.

Dry Drunk: Behave as if drunk or hungover, but not having had anything to drink at all. Often shows as a loss of previous serenity, which is replaced by angry mood swings, return of tension and perfectionism, being over-critical of others, being childish and demanding, etc.

Emotional involvement or dependency: Falling in love, being infatuated, unwilling to spend time away from the particular person, day-dreaming about him or her, sexual fantasies involving him or her.

Intellectualising: Using brain power to produce rationalisations and defences. Obscure straightforward simple things with complications.

Manipulative: Always try to arrange things to suit yourself.

Personal maturity: Having adult attitudes.

Personality: Character; manner in which a person deals with life.

Sadness: Feeling of depression, unhappiness, low energy, often the mask for inner anger which isn't shown because of lack of assertiveness.

Sponsor: Person of same sex in AA whom you can trust and who guides you in early sobriety.

Tension: Feeling of being uptight, strained, on edge, restless, can't relax.

CHAPTER 8

Staying sober and the dangers of being a Dry Drunk

If you have decided to stop drinking because there were problems in your life from alcohol (Chapter 1) and you decided you were alcoholic (Chapter 2) you were advised that the only safe course is to stay stopped altogether. To the non-addict this is no problem — it is a rational decision, and no other factors interfere with it.

> I was getting these terrible stomach pains. The doctor did an X-ray and told me I had a stomach ulcer. He said I needed to take some special pills, watch my diet — and no alcohol. I followed his instructions, and I've been perfectly well since.

It is never so easy for the addict. In Chapter 7, attitudes that make it easy to start drinking again such as complacency, feelings and emotions, guilt and depression were described. To guard against these things, you must struggle to introduce an attitude change into your whole lifestyle. The Alcoholics Anonymous Programme is one way of getting support, keeping with the winners and developing your sense of spirituality.

Some AA slogans are particularly helpful;

> One day at a time.
> Think, think, think.
> Let Go and Let God.
> First things first.
> Is it really important?

Expect to have mood swings, and guard against the sudden bad day, when giving up alcohol does not seem worth it. That is when you must not be alone, but find a straight friend to talk to. Do not go and see your old drinking or pot-smoking friends — they will not be helpful in keeping your sobriety.

An often quoted slogan is HALT, reminding you to avoid:
   H — Hunger
   A — Aggression or anger
   L — Love or new emotional entanglements, or Loneliness
   T — Tiredness
These things all increase stress: something you want to minimise in early sobriety.

Remember it takes something like two years to incorporate change into our lives on an enduring basis, so this is a good length of time to aim at following instructions without cutting corners. Alas, so many alcoholics are impatient, and want to run before they can walk, getting cross when told, 'Easy does it!'

Anti-alcohol pills

The drugs Antabuse and Dipsan are white pills that look like aspirin, and work in the liver (not the brain). They are not mind-changing; instead, they block the breakdown of alcohol and cause nausea, vomiting, headaches and low blood pressure, if someone drinks while taking them.

> I was on Antabuse, and felt low, so I thought, 'What the hell', and went into the nearest pub and had a triple Scotch. Nothing much happened, so I had another. Then, after about 15 minutes I suddenly felt violently ill. My head was splitting, I couldn't get my breath. Someone called an ambulance and I went to Accident and Emergency. Sure works okay. Stopped me going on a bender.

Antabuse or Dipsan do not stop craving. They just make you ill if you drink. Their main use is to reinforce your decision that, just for today, you are not going to drink. If you take them in the morning, you know that whatever happens and however you feel for the rest of that day, you will not be able to drink. Never mind next week or next year — *today* you are not drinking. Families often visibly relax once they see their alcoholic willingly taking Antabuse. You must take it because you want to demonstrate *you* do not want to drink. Otherwise you could be like the chap in this story.

> My wife used to insist I took Antabuse each morning. She could
> not understand how I could drink on them. She called the doctor
> all sorts of names. But she did not know I had changed the pills
> in the bottle for aspirins!

To keep sober, obviously you need to remain honest!

The correct dose of either Antabuse or Dipsan should be
determined by your doctor. They can only be obtained on prescription. An effective dose is usually a tablet per day, but
sometimes two tablets per day are necessary.

Antabuse has been in use since the 1950s, and is remark-
ably safe. However, it should not be taken during pregnancy
(neither should any other drug, including alcohol). Sometimes
it causes bad breath, and/or a metallic taste in the mouth. The
dose should be reduced if this happens. Amplex tablets, obtainable from chemists without prescription, may also help. Ask
your spouse if your breath smells, because people don't
usually like to comment — but bad breath can be difficult to
live with. Sometimes Antabuse makes people tired. Usually
this passes off in a few days, but if it persists, take Antabuse
at bed time, and turn this side-effect to good use. About one
in a million people may have other rare side-effects, about
which doctors argue, such as peripheral neuritis (see page 10)
and crazy thinking patterns. I have seen one case of the latter
in 16 years — it is completely reversible. Some doctors will
not give Antabuse where there is severe liver damage — but
often the liver damage is so severe in these cases that it acts
as its own deterrent.

Every medically used drug has drawbacks. Even penicillin
kills people (through sensitivity reactions) as well as curing
countless others. Antabuse is as safe or safer than penicillin.
You must decide whether the relief of knowing you can't
drink for the day is worth running the slight risk of a side-
effect (and just think of the side-effects of alcohol if you are
still not convinced . . .).

> When John came home, I know I didn't trust him. It was a relief
> to me to see him taking Antabuse of his own free will every day.
> I knew then he was serious, and that he was backing up his
> promises with action. I'd get tense each month as his prescrip-

tion ran down, I'd ask myself if he'd get another or not. After three months of this, he noticed what was happening and talked to me about it. I think that conversation really helped our relationship. I could see how much he'd changed. And he got three-monthly repeats from our doctor after that.

My advice is to take Antabuse for two years because, as already mentioned, this is the average time it takes to get used to new behaviour in your life.

Being a Dry Drunk

'Dry Drunks' are sober people whose behaviour is as bad as when they were drinking. Their loved ones may suddenly explode with 'You were easier to live with when you were drinking!' Sometimes a recovering alcoholic is so pleased with himself that his ego is over-inflated and his wife can't stand him, as in this situation:

> John seemed to think I should congratulate him every day because he was sober. As if he'd done something really clever and wanted a pat on the head, like our little boy. And yet all he'd done was decide to live in the normal world. I don't see why I need to praise him up for that.

Dry Drunks may be seen by their friends as some of the following: arrogant, 'up themselves', aggressive, taking others for granted, tense and over-striving, over-ambitious, complacent about their alcoholism, quick to lose their temper, selfish or self-centred, avoiding old friends or having a change in their sleeping pattern. Sometimes it is like one long BUD (page 54) without the physical craving for alcohol. Being a Dry Drunk interferes with relationships, and therefore with your quality of life, so if you realise you are acting like a Dry Drunk, talk it out with your sponsor and your local alcoholism counsellor and consider both outpatient and inpatient therapy. If untreated, Dry Drunks tend to become wet ones!

Lastly, I have to laugh about some folk who come saying they are Dry Drunks, but when I get an accurate history of the past few months, I find there is the odd drink, the odd pill, or the odd smoke of cannabis. I cannot repeat often enough that for the alcoholic, taking any mind-changing drug constitutes an end to sobriety. Such people are not Dry Drunks at all. They have reactivated their chemical addiction and they are, for our purposes, Wet Drunks — no self-deception, please! (The only exception to this is the prescription by a doctor of specific antidepressant medication — see Chapter 16.)

Sometimes Dry Drunk behaviour is a signal of clinical depression, and this needs treatment in its own right. Depression sometimes appears for the first time three to six months after getting sober, often as the full impact of what has been going on actually dawns on the person. Signs are: waking early in the morning; unable to get back to sleep; ruminating on guilt; unable to shake off black thoughts; feeling that life is pointless, not worth the struggle; loss of appetite; loss of weight; constipation; sense of doom and dread that things will never be better; suicidal thoughts; feeling of contaminating others with own badness. If you are depressed talk to your friends, counsellor or doctor. Don't wallow in guilt or self-pity!

Things you can do

1 Do you have a good balance between work and play?
2 Are you developing or finding new ways of having fun which are appropriate for your age, degree of physical fitness, talents, new ideals, new desires?
3 Should you be taking Antabuse?
4 Read the 'Dry Drunk' pamphlet obtainable from AA General Service Office, PO Box 6458, Wellington, New Zealand.
5 If you find yourself 'thinking drinking' you are in a BUD. Talk it out with a trusted friend or your AA sponsor, by phone or in person — but do it quickly before events overtake you. Remind yourself of the bad things that have happened to you as a result of drinking. Do not focus on the happy times. One man I know kept a card in his wallet with the dates of his separations from his wife, his appearance in court for driving while intoxicated, and the date of his entry to Queen Mary Hospital. He looked at it whenever he found himself wanting to drink.

Key words

Antabuse; Abstem: Two drugs that stop the breakdown of alcohol in the liver, causing vomiting, headache and other unpleasant effects about 15–30 minutes after drinking booze.

Attitude change: Change the way you react to the things that happen to you.

Craving: Urgent desire to drink or take drugs. Dangerous time for alcoholics/addicts.

Dry Drunk: Behave as if drunk or hungover, but not having had anything to drink at all. Often shows as a loss of previous serenity, which is replaced by angry mood swings, return of tension and perfectionism, being over-critical of others, being childish and demanding, etc.

Inebriation: Another word for being drunk — introduced to try to indicate the effects of being drunk without the degrading overtones of the word 'drunk'.

Mood swings: Sudden changes from being happy to being sad; from serenity to anger; from acceptance to complacency. Sign of immaturity or childishness.

Stress: Feeling of having too much to cope with, too much on your plate.

Over-inflated ego: A term for somebody who thinks and acts like a 'big shot'; usually associated with a chip on the shoulder; thinks the world revolves around him or her (usually him). Mask for insecurity.

CHAPTER 9
Alcoholic brain damage

In recent years it has been possible to take special X-rays of the brain that show if there is tissue shrinkage. A large number of living alcoholics have now been examined in this way. The results show that approximately 90 per cent of chronic alcoholics have brain shrinkage. It recovers slowly over about two years, but not always completely. At present there are no sensitive tests for measuring early mental changes, but as the damage progresses, the following become more obvious:

- Poor memory — forget appointments, shopping lists, can't retain new information.
- Harder to learn new skills.
- Concentration not as good — mind wanders when reading a book or following a complicated speaker.
- Find it hard to solve new problems or cope with situations.
- Go to pieces under stress — lose temper, or get very tense and perform badly.

Alcoholic brain damage is different from that caused by knocks to the head, or strokes (which are caused either by bleeding into the brain or loss of blood supply because of thrombosis). These other types of brain damage result in difficulties in speaking and movement of limbs. This does not usually happen in alcoholic brain damage. Alcoholics with quite damaged functioning can talk the hind leg off a donkey if they could do so before — there is no problem with words

— and they can also run and jump just as well — some groups in the United States even have AA Olympics. Rather than affecting speech or the movement of limbs, alcoholic brain damage affects the powers of concentration, memory and temper control, and it is now known that the more brain damage that is present, the more likely it is that relapse will occur.

How can you tell if you have alcoholic brain damage? First, compare your performance after six weeks of *total* abstinence to your known performance before you started drinking. Make some allowance for the passing years. If you know your concentration is poor, you forget things, you lose your temper more easily, take criticism harder — then the chances are that your brain is damaged.

Second, you can ask your doctor or counsellor to arrange special tests.

Third, it is realistic to assume that if you have exceeded the levels given in Figure 1 (page 6) for two to five years, then some brain damage will have occurred. My prediction is that as we develop better tests, we are going to show earlier and earlier brain damage. Young people are just as liable to have it as old people.

Fourth, there are some other symptoms that may be present:

- Withdrawal fits — an epileptic seizure brought on by drop in blood alcohol level.
- More frequent alcoholic 'blackouts', better called 'blank-outs', when you walk and talk normally but later have absolutely no memory of what happened.
- Developing the very serious medical conditions of Wernicke's Syndrome (altered state of consciousness, eye squint, unsteady walk) or Korsakoff's Psychosis (can't remember anything new ever again, make up stories to explain events, need mental hospital care. It's a bit late if you've got this — cure is rare, improvement very slow).

Things you can do

1 Decide if you have brain damage — reread the five symptoms on page 65.
2 If so, get plenty of support, avoid stress, avoid getting too

ambitious. Stick close to AA. Take it seriously — it won't
go away!

3 Remain totally abstinent from all mind-changing chemicals
— cannabis (pot), valium and all other minor tranquillisers
can also cause brain damage. Remind yourself that recovery in brain function goes on for at least two years, possibly
a lot longer. Even one drink may jeopardise this process.

4 Eat a balanced diet to ensure a healthy vitamin intake.
Multi-vitamin tablets are unnecessary if you eat properly
and are abstinent, unless your doctor recommends them after checking your blood.

5 Learn to accept yourself and, while it is healthy to grieve
the past, self-pity is quite unhelpful. See life as a challenge.
If you react to stress by losing your temper, take Step 10
of the AA programme: 'Continued to take personal inventory, and when we were wrong, promptly admitted it.'

Key words

Alcoholic brain damage: When the brain has been damaged by
alcohol, causing problems with concentration, memory, and
keeping temper.

Balanced diet: 'Diet' is the food you eat every day. 'Balanced'
means containing a balance of all types of food: protein (e.g.,
eggs, cheese, meat, fish), carbohydrates (e.g., bread, potatoes,
rice), fat, fresh fruit and vegetables — i.e., 'proper' food, not
just fast food or junk food!

Relapse: Start drinking again after deciding to be sober.

Withdrawal fits, 'Rum' fits, epileptic seizures: Whatever the
cause, all fits look the same: a fall to the ground (sometimes
resulting in injury), a brief cry, a loss of consciousness, jerking
movements and difficulty in breathing. May last a few minutes
only, followed by minutes or hours of sleepiness. All fits are
frightening for bystanders but the patient won't remember that
he has had one.

CHAPTER 10

Women and addiction: special facts

With equality of the sexes, women are learning to drink like men. Women are also the target of much advertising (especially for wine) because they represent an underdeveloped market to sellers of booze. More and more women will have alcohol problems because of this increase in drinking. While a woman with an alcohol problem has the same sort of symptoms as a man, there are certain important differences, as follows.

Women's bodies and brains get damaged more quickly than men's, for an equal amount of alcohol. This is because women are generally lighter than men, and because more of their body weight is made up of fat. When alcohol is absorbed into the body, it is distributed everywhere via the blood vessels. Fat has fewer blood vessels than other body tissue, so alcohol is more quickly distributed elsewhere. The other tissues therefore get a high level of alcohol in them, and more direct damage. The old wives' tale that women get drunk more easily than men is therefore quite true.

Women also get liver damage more quickly than men because of this process. Tissue damage caused by alcohol is always dose-related. The higher the dose, the greater the damage.

Because of the traditional place of women in the home, their lives are very closely linked to those of their husbands. If he is a drinker, they will drink too. Many women report that this is how their addiction began. Also, a woman whose work is mainly in the home is able to drink secretly, and often her family will cover up for her. This is related to the stigma attached to being a woman alcoholic, and this feeling of shame may prevent help being sought. For some reason, society seems to consider that a woman alcoholic is 'worse' than a male alcoholic, an attitude that results in women feeling disadvantaged in legal disputes involving separation and custody of children. This is unfortunate, because in my experience women do better than men in therapy because they are more prepared to talk about their emotions.

Alcohol in pregnancy

Women alcoholics who drink heavily during pregnancy can damage their babies. The damage occurs because alcohol crosses from the mother's blood through the placenta (afterbirth) into the baby. The most dangerous time is during early and mid-pregnancy, when the brain is developing fast. One effect of alcohol is to produce a less intelligent child, even sometimes to cause a child to develop such a low IQ that it is intellectually handicapped. Some children have a particular facial appearance, consisting of narrowed eye openings, short upturned nose, flat cheeks, short head width, thin upper lip and wide mouth. All this is called Foetal Alcohol Syndrome.

Of course children born into alcoholic families are going to be brought up affected by the alcoholic behaviour of mother, so it is hard to know what behaviours are caused by brain damage to the baby, and which are learned as the child grows up. See Chapter 15, page 102 — Adult Children of Alcoholics.

It is not known exactly how much alcohol will cause Foetal Alcohol Syndrome. The only safe dose is nothing during pregnancy. Obviously the heavier the dose, the greater likelihood of damage. One study suggested that half the children of women drinking 150 grams of alcohol per day (equivalent to six bottles of beer, two bottles of wine or half a bottle of spirits) had severely affected children.

Marijuana (cannabis) is also thought to produce a similar syndrome to alcohol. It may well be that sleeping pills and minor tranquillisers (e.g., Valium, Mogadon, Ativan, Rohypnol,

Imovane) do this too. Although the scientific evidence is lacking at the time of writing, in principle they act in the same way.

Social issues for women

The position of women in society is traditionally less powerful than that of men. Women have great pressure on them to be homemakers and mothers first, and career people second. Women are expected to get married, not to play around before marriage, and to surrender to their husband's will and needs. The women's liberation movement of the past hundred years is attempting to change this, but the fact is that our world is still mostly male dominated. New Zealand has a long history of promoting female equality. For instance, we were the first country in the world to grant women the vote (in 1893). But you only have to count the female members of Parliament to get a clear idea of how male dominated our system of government remains. There is a long way to go before power is shared between the sexes.

What does this mean in relation to women's alcohol or drug taking? Often it means there is a strong feeling of powerlessness, of being second all the time, of not really being worth much, of being easily forced to conform to the wishes of others (particularly men). If you have read right through this book to this point, you will immediately see how these feelings will produce resentment and low self-esteem. These feelings are often the seedbed of chemical addiction. Drugs produce temporary relief but do nothing to solve the basic problem, thus it is easy to seek more relief through drugs, and so on into addiction.

> When I got married, I felt I'd given up something that was good
> [an office job] and taken up something not so good. Before I had
> my own money and could spend it how I liked. Suddenly I had
> none, except what my husband gave me. There wasn't much left
> after he'd been to the pub and the TAB. It got worse after the
> children were born. I thought if he drank, I might as well too.

Women have been in this position for many years, even centuries, so what has changed that results in more alcohol and drug taking? I think the answer is more money and changing expectations. In Victorian times the choice was often between food or alcohol. Mothers hated booze because it literally caused starvation. The Temperance Alliance had thousands of members because of this, and almost brought in prohibition of alcohol in 1918. Our welfare state today ensures children and families don't starve when a parent becomes alcoholic, so this makes it easier for people to drink. There is more money around, and women (quite rightly) are no longer content to play second fiddle to male domination. If there is more disappointment or losses, there will be more resentment, and hence the likelihood of relief drinking. (See Chapter 6, page 45.)

Difficulties faced by women who want to recover

Many of the particular difficulties faced by women who want to recover are related to the social issue discussed above. Thus women feel more stigmatised because 'mother should be responsible'. (Watch out for those *shoulds* in recovery — they often further reduce our self-esteem, and make us feel hopeless or a failure.) As a result, women tend to deny their addiction for longer. Women find it harder to get therapy because of child-care responsibilities.

> Ann had been in treatment at Queen Mary Hospital as both an addict and a co-dependent for two weeks, when her alcoholic husband rang her up to tell her, very angrily, she should come home and look after the children. Coached by the staff, she told him the children were his responsibility as much as hers and she needed therapy for herself. He threatened to get a plane and a rental car and dump the children at the hospital. Ann's doctor then intervened, to tell the husband that care could be arranged for the children, to allow him to come to Family Week at the hospital, and discuss the problem he and Ann were facing. He rang off angrily. Next day, Ann's doctor telephoned again — and he had agreed.

Women employed in jobs in traditionally male-dominated fields tend to drink and smoke more, presumably related to the stress of competition. Psychiatric research suggests that depression and suicide attempts are more clearly linked to alcoholism in women than in men.

The guilt women feel about their powerlessness over their

addiction and the effect it has on their families, is often greater than men's. Some Swedish research suggests that alcoholic mothers are more likely to have daughters and sons who become alcoholic, whereas fathers tend to hand on their alcoholism to sons only.

Women who have a clear premenstrual syndrome (PMT) do tend to overuse alcohol and drugs, so this is an additional hurdle. However, surveys of women alcoholics indicate only about a quarter have PMT. It is part of male-dominated attitudes to insist that all women suffer from PMT and a clear fact is that most do not.

Gay women (lesbians) face the stigma of both sexual orientation and alcoholism/addiction. There is a welcome trend towards tolerance of both men's and women's sexual orientation, but prejudice and misunderstanding affect a lot of people. Shame or guilt are often severe, especially in the children of dysfunctional families, who have not been taught how to deal with them. Lesbian women have a high incidence of alcohol and drug problems, presumably because of feelings of alienation, isolation and relationship problems. Recovery demands a high degree of openness, acceptance of support, and vigorous honesty in processing feelings and conducting relationships.

Women have a higher incidence of sexual abuse, both in childhood and adult life, than men. This is frequently linked to gynaecological problems and sexual dysfunction in later life. The sexual area of our lives rarely gets talked about openly, and this will be even less likely if you come from a dysfunctional background, or if you feel powerless. In recovery, ask for information (presumably that is why you are reading this book!), and process your feelings with women you trust.

13th stepping

In AA and NA, people are encouraged to get a sponsor — a person you can trust who is in recovery. You are encouraged to telephone, consult with and be advised by this person on a daily basis, rather than go off alone or back to friends who are still using, and risk reactivating your addiction. Clearly, you can get quite attached to your sponsor. This relationship will cease to be helpful if it becomes sexual. Thus, males are told to have male sponsors, and females to have female sponsors — avoid cross-sex sponsorship always. The only exception to this is in the case of homosexual people: total honesty and openness are necessary here. The ideals of the Twelve Steps of AA and NA are beyond reproach, but ideals are not always followed by human beings, who sometimes make mistakes. The phrase '13th stepping' has been coined to remind us that this step is *not* part of the AA programme. See also Chapter 13, pages 97.

Eating disorders

More and more women who drink excessively are revealing problems with pills, dieting and weight control. Such women often have low self-esteem, a feeling of insecurity, and chronic fear of not meeting standards they set themselves. This perfectionism extends to being 'the right shape', sometimes with disastrous results.

> My thighs and hips were just too large. I cried and cried because there was nothing I could do about it, until I learned about dieting.

The 19-year-old who said this was the only child of an alcoholic father and the classic co-dependent mother (see Chapter 12). Her home life revolved around Dad's binge drinking. No wonder she was insecure and immature. There was even a suspicion of a sexual relationship between daughter and father (see page 106).

Another alcoholic with weight control problems had this to say:

> My dieting started when I was 20. I changed from being a chubby teenager to what I thought was a very elegant shape. I felt very tired all the time, and I began to drink to give myself energy. I took laxatives and diuretics to keep slim — easy to get because I was a nurse — and really puzzled the doctors my family sent me to. I had two disastrous marriages, both to alcoholics, and went on drinking, pill popping and eating binges.

Behind the preoccupation with externals like body shape lies an insecure person, with overpowering feelings which are poorly recognised and expressed. Recovery occurs with the recognition of inner feelings, and linking these to eating or drugging. Keeping an emotional diary often helps, providing that there is trust between patient and counsellor.

> My therapist insisted I write down the events preceding each binge. Gradually it dawned on me how something triggered each episode. Writing it down helped me express it and I felt less trapped. I still have the odd time when I relapse, but I don't feel it is the end of the world, and when I do, I look for what has caused me to feel so low. I go and talk to my friends, or make an appointment with my therapist, or attend a psychodrama group.

Psychodrama is a method of therapy involving acting through our feelings. It enables us to experience how others see us, and this helps to adjust to reality. Eating disorders are often, but not always, mixed with drug or alcohol dependency. They always represent a severe communication difficulty, and such sufferers need a lot of help to develop healthier ways of expressing their feelings, needs and wants. Incidentally, more men are developing problems with food and beginning to talk about them in therapy groups.

Things you can do

1 If you are a female alcoholic, do you feel 'worse', more ashamed, than male alcoholics? It is important to relieve yourself of these guilty feelings. Try talking to other female recovering alcoholics (e.g., at AA meetings or local AA centre if you live in a city). Try talking to a female counsellor at the local Alcohol and Drug Centre. Try doing steps 4 and 5 of the AA programme (see Chapter 6).

2 How do you rate your own self-worth? Write down ten good things about yourself. We all have good and bad points — your self-assessment needs to be realistic if you are going to recover from alcoholism.

3 Make amends to people you've hurt, except where to do so would cause further harm (steps 8 and 9 of the AA programme). This relieves shame and guilt.

4 If you tend to overeat, keep a diary of events, thoughts, and emotions that precede your binge. Does overeating follow particular experiences?

5 Is your eating problem more serious, e.g., do you vomit purposely when you have eaten a lot? Are you very overweight? Try contacting Overeaters Anonymous (see page 146 for address).

6 Your own doctor or the local Alcohol and Drug Centre will be able to tell you where you can get expert help locally.

7 Read *Our Shout: Women and Alcohol*, by Helen Warren, Chris Griffiths and Ingrid Huygens, Heinemann Reed, 1989.

Key words

Alcoholic hepatitis: Inflammation of the liver caused by alcohol. Can lead on to cirrhosis.

Cirrhosis: Liver damage caused by the death of liver cells from alcohol poisoning. Luckily not all the liver is killed at the same time — it is usually a gradual process over many years, and can be arrested by sobriety.

Emotional diary: Keeping a daily written account of how you are feeling, then using this to see what the link is between drinking (or taking drugs, or eating excessively) and emotions.

Psychodrama: Group therapy method of examining life problems by acting them through, not just talking about them. Easier to understand how it helps by attending a demonstration session. Most main centres in New Zealand offer occasional groups.

CHAPTER 11

Alcoholism, chemical dependency and being Maori

The impact of European culture on the traditional Maori way of life since the early 1800s has left many Maori people with a feeling of being different and not belonging either to Maoridom or to European culture.

> I have always tried to be a dark-skinned Pakeha. I suppose I am ashamed of being Maori.

> My father wouldn't teach me Maori. He told me to learn the Pakeha ways because that was the world I'd have to live in.

And this, said by a middle-aged person:

> At school we were given the strap if we spoke Maori. I learned to keep quiet about what my nana taught me. I feel as if I carry all the old knowledge inside me. It's going to die with me (weeps). It is such a burden.

The definition of being Maori is simple: if you feel Maori, no matter how small your blood line, then you are Maori. The opposite applies too: if you feel European, then you are European, no matter how big your blood line. This immediately means we must be honest with ourselves. Such self-honesty isn't always easy. In this book it has often been recommended that you should talk out complicated feelings with people you trust.

This chapter is co-authored with Mrs Monica Stockdale, director of the Taha Maori Programme at Queen Mary Hospital, Hanmer Springs.

> My therapist at Queen Mary Hospital asked me if I was Maori.
> I said I was, but I didn't want to have anything to do with the
> other Maoris at the hospital. She told me if I wanted to stay at the
> hospital I'd have to go to four sessions of the group. At first I
> resisted, but as soon as I walked into the Wharenui, I felt I'd
> come home. I felt very ashamed that I'd cut myself off from my
> heritage, my culture. I felt like crying when they began to sing
> the waiata. It was like being back in a happy family, my whanau,
> only without the violence and abuse.

This speaker refers to the joy of returning to the best of
Maoridom, without the violence and abuse. He was the victim
of sexual abuse while a child, accompanied by threats of
violence and, occasionally, severe beatings. This disadvantaged background is all too common in both Maori men and
women, especially where there is a family history of alcoholism. Such people are called adult children of alcoholics (see
Chapter 15). When bad things happen during our upbringing,
we often react to them without realising it.

> All my life I've been violent. I have verbally abused my wife. I've
> hit her too. I feel so ashamed . . . and guilty. My nana taught me
> that was bad. But how could I tell her that one of my brothers
> was sexually abusing me? I had nowhere to turn. Mum and Dad
> didn't know what was happening — they were back home and I
> was with Nana. I ran off one day to find my way home, but a
> neighbour brought me home, and I got a thrashing from Grandad.

When a child isn't heard, the unfairness of it all can result
in resentments that set the stage for alcohol and drug problems later on. Often this process is added to that of separation
from Maoridom, resulting in a big dose of alienation and
despair. Such feelings are often covered up with violence in
men, and promiscuity in women.

At Queen Mary Hospital, when Maori people attend the
Taha Maori programme they often suddenly realise that this is
where they belong, even if they have no knowledge of Maoritanga. They set about learning, and find this is a way to heal
their feelings of despair and loss. These are spiritual feelings,
or wairua, and once they are allowed to flow, they will result in
a rekindling of connections with our ancestors (tupuna), the
earth (Papatuanuku and mauri) and finally result in a 'place

where we can stand' (turangawaewae).

Maori who are alcoholic and chemically addicted need all the other things in this book, plus establishing their sense of identity. The ability of Maori to care for each other (manaki-tanga) with love (aroha) adds greatly to the wairua and mana of each, and increases the chance of recovery. Time and again staff members have been deeply moved to see addicts who have been cut off from themselves for years, develop a sense of identity and purpose within the hospital whanau (family). This helps them start on their journey towards wholeness and healing. Sometimes the love and support (awhi) offered amongst Maori has led to jealousy from Pakeha who do not have such a recent cultural heritage to call on.

Until Europeans came to Aotearoa, the Maori people did not drink alcohol. By all accounts, the conduct of the early sailors amounted to drunken debauchery, but as time went on, this situation reversed itself, with succeeding waves of European immigrants being of more sober habits and Maori becoming heavier drinkers. Some historians consider this early training in heavy drinking by sailors seeking 'rest and recreation' was very significant in setting the new customs for drinking.

In Maori tribal life alcohol was only occasionally available, because there was little to make it from. Alcohol is fermented from starch — like potatoes, corn, and sugar. Maori grew kumara, but not in large enought amounts to have much left over for conversion to alcohol. Tutu berries were sometimes collected and fermented, but only at certain times of the year, in small quantities. No other form of starch was available. Cannabis was unknown also. When European sailors began bringing alcohol ashore in the early 1800s, this was soon followed by potatoes and wheat growing. Maori quickly adopted these new methods and were supplying the settlers with food, and making money doing this. This extra money could be converted to alcohol, and set the stage for heavy drinking.

CHAPTER 12

Co-dependency (1):
For wives married to alcoholic husbands

The word *co-dependency* describes the lifestyle of those who live with a person who is dependent on alcohol or other drugs. What follows is written specifically for the wife of a male alcoholic, but the same principles apply to the husband of a female alcoholic, or to the spouse of any chemically dependent person, although obviously the details are different. Some gender differences are dealt with in Chapter 14, and suggestions that other family members (children, friends, parents) can follow are outlined in Chapter 15. If drugs (cannabis, opiates, minor tranquillisers) are the main problem in your circumstances, this chapter will still be helpful for you if you substitute 'addiction' and 'addicted person' for 'alcoholism' and 'alcoholic' as you read through.

Alcoholism is a sickness, and living with an alcoholic husband gradually makes a wife sick too. This sickness consists of:

- Denial that your beloved really is an alcoholic.
- Rows over why he keeps drinking.
- Organising the family so life goes on around the drinking.
- Increasing feelings of being powerless to change things.
- Efforts to protect your children.

Living with an alcoholic trains you to react in certain ways. This training is of course unhealthy, and is how you 'catch' the sickness of co-dependency. The first step in recovery is to decide you are powerless over your alcoholic. This means you need to realise you cannot ever make him get better. If he wants to recover, then he will. The only way that you can help is to ensure that he feels the consequences of his addiction: after all, if you bang you head against a brick wall it hurts, and so you stop your banging. Ensure he sees his own messes 'the morning after'. Ensure he answers the phone call from the boss himself, pays the household bills himself. If you go out to work, be sure you sit down together first and decide what you are going to do with your money. Otherwise you will find you are paying for the food, rates, clothes and so on while he just has extra booze money. This is a prime example of 'enabling' (see Key words). Another is keeping the children quiet because he has a hangover, or 'walking on eggshells' so as not to upset him.

Many wives get very resentful that the alcoholic seems to have all the power to do as he likes, while they have to be dogs-body and doormat. In recovery for the co-dependent, you will learn that you will be happiest if you sidestep fights, but do not surrender your power. This is the subtle approach of *tough love*. Love him enough to let him feel the consequences of his addiction. You will only be able to do this if you deal with your own denial first. Have you faced the situation squarely?

A recovering alcoholic once told me:

> I remember I came home from the pub about 8 p.m., and nobody was at home. I was worried. Where *was* Jenny? She came back at 10 p.m. and I called her all sorts of names. I remember being surprised when she didn't react. Told me she'd been out with some women friends to a Church Hall.
>
> 'I suppose you've been bitching about your husbands, as usual,' I said.
>
> She replied, 'I'm really anxious about Justin' (that's our son), 'he needs a new tyre for his bike. Could you get one tomorrow?' Then she went to bed.
>
> I had a feeling something had really changed in her. I didn't know then what it was. I know now she'd been to Al-Anon and had started to work the programme. She went every week and it was some time before she told me where she was going. I was really angry when I found out. I laugh about it now. But she defused it by saying she wasn't going there for me, but for her-

self. Well, life had been easier between us, so I didn't have a leg
to stand on.

This is the early stage of tough love, where the co-dependent
wife begins to sidestep fights, and to care for herself in a helpful way. She is changing her negative coping responses and
her sense of powerlessness into more positive responses.

Examples of *negative coping responses* which do *not* help
you or him, but which keep you fighting about the wrong
things in the wrong way are:

- Hitting him, showing him up in public.
- Having rows about his drinking; being a nagging wife.
- Feeling too hopeless/helpless to do anything, so give up.
- Keeping away when he is drinking. Becoming bitter.
- Giving him booze money. Cleaning up after him.
- Giving him alcohol to help withdrawals.
- Searching for hidden bottles. Pouring away supplies.
- Pretending all is well to friends, the doctor, etc.
- Going out to work to pay bills; drinking with him so he
  doesn't get so drunk.
- Smoothing over his troubles with others, e.g., employers.
- Doing anything to avoid a fight, e.g., submitting to degrad-
  ing sex.
- Threatening to leave.
- Hating the thought of going home.
- Locking him out of the house.
- Getting drunk yourself.
- Becoming dependent on tranquillisers or anti-depressants.

Alcoholics often say, 'If you were married to my wife,
you'd drink too, Doc!' They mean they live with behaviour
like that listed above. However, such behaviour is the result
of living with alcoholism, not the cause of it. In the course of
meeting hundreds of wives of alcoholics, I categorically state
that I have *never* come across a single case where the wife
drove the husband to drink! Modern research points to the
fact that there is no such things as a typical wife of an alcoholic. Wives are normal people reacting to the stress of living
with alcoholism, and trying to cope with it. In trying to cope
they often find themselves doing the same things as other
wives in the same situation.

Instead, you should try to introduce *positive coping responses* into your life. The principle is to create an independent existence for yourself within the marriage, to safeguard your own happiness. This is not abandoning him, but is recognising that his alcoholism (over which you have no control, remember, and neither, due to his denial, has he) is a selfish disease. Until his denial cracks, there is nothing you can do except safeguard your own sanity by:

- Arranging social activities, friends of your own.
- Going out with a girlfriend to the films if he never takes you. (You can get babysitters if you try.)
- Taking up new hobbies.
- Going out to Al-Anon and following the programme. (A similar group, Nar-Anon, exists for families of chemically dependent people, but is not fully developed everywhere in New Zealand yet.)
- Getting a job (but make sure that this doesn't just give him extra booze money).
- Avoiding fights about the wrong things.
- Practising honesty in communication.
- Never making a bogus threat.
- Never talking to him about serious matters when he is drunk — wait until he is sober.
- Making sure he cleans up his own messes, within reason.
- Planning a refuge if you fear physical violence, e.g., going to your mother's, a friend's, or perhaps the Women's Refuge if there is one. The Salvation Army always tries to help. Some New Zealand cities may have an Al-Anon 'safe' home — get the address from your local Al-Anon Group, which will be in the telephone book.

Examples of positive coping responses

Him: alcoholic's behaviour	Her: positive coping response
Arrives late for tea from the pub regularly.	Tell him what time his tea will be ready. Dish it up, place it in the oven and leave it there. If it frizzles up, it frizzles up. That is the consequence of being late.

	Do not pretend otherwise or be a martyr or insist he be there. It is his choice. Keep calm.
Has not paid electricity and it is to be cut off.	Allow it to be cut off. Ask him what he intends to do about it. We survived before electricity.
Hits you.	This is a time for *serious* action. Move out the next day to a friendly base. No woman should ever put up with this. Negotiate terms of return, e.g., that he has treatment.
Is cruel to the children.	Say nothing (within reason) because you are probably being 'set up'. But how can you stay when this is happening? Wait until he is sober. Sit him down. Tell him what he did and what your limits are. Never make a threat you won't carry out, but conversely don't put up with rubbish. Plan your retreat to a friendly base (as above).
Crashes the car — gets drunk in charge *or* Rapes you *or* Vomits blood *or* Has withdrawals *or* Loses job through drinking.	These are all examples of a *crisis*. Make sure that you *use* the crisis to assist him in getting sober. Move out to a friendly base and insist he goes to alcoholism counsellor as condition of living together. See doctor with him and be clear about his alcohol intake to ensure drinking does not remain secret. Attend Al-Anon and Family Counselling Centre or local Alcohol and Drug Centre yourself.
He comes home after work every day, turns on the TV, has a few drinks, has tea and goes back to TV and some more	Treat your husband's drinking problem as *serious*. This isn't the marriage you planned together. Talk to him when he is sober

drink, then sleeps from 8 p.m. onwards. He never hits you or argues, but is quite passive. May be quite open about drinking or be a secret drinker. You are married to a zombie.

and not tired, e.g., Saturday morning. If no improvement, plan an active life which takes you out to Al-Anon, and your friends. Remember the unhappiest people are those with no friends. Await a crisis (as above). If none occurs, consider Family Members' Programme admission for yourself.

You know he isn't the man he was because of drinking, but there are violent arguments whenever alcohol is brought up.

Stop fighting over the wrong issues: his denial prevents him from being rational. Plan independent life; learn about Al-Anon; await a crisis.

He tells you repeatedly that he drinks because you are a nagging wife/on his back/a worrier/an old misery-guts/hopeless with money/a useless bitch, etc.

If he tells you something often enough you may start to believe him. Therefore be sure you have some friends away from him who can appreciate your true worth. Do not let the disease ruin your self-esteem as it has ruined his!

Don't become a mother to your alcoholic

Because of feelings of powerlessness, and fears of retaliation, many women are unable or afraid to set limits to their alcoholic's behaviour. You will have to make you own decision about what is reasonable for you to put up with, and what is not. This is where a discussion with your local alcoholism counsellor, and attendance at Al-Anon will help.

Many women have had childhoods where they learned to be powerless. This may include being the child in an alcoholic family (see Chapter 15), or being sexually abused, or abused in other ways. To change that requires personal awareness and personal growth. As mentioned on page 40, this cannot happen from reading books, unfortunately. You learn it in therapy groups, in counselling, or in Al-Anon, or sometimes in talking to your friends, if you have got the right ones. Be courageous and learn to talk about your inner feelings to people you can trust.

After I went to see the counsellor at my local Alcohol and Drug Centre, I realised I didn't just have two young children, I had a grown-up one as well. It was like a flash of light, realising that Garry was behaving like a child in many respects, because of his alcoholism. Once I expected him to behave like that, instead of kidding myself he was putting it on, a lot of the heat went out of our relationship. Now I'm waiting for a crisis when I can act. It won't be long coming because I am refusing to take responsibility for the effects of his addiction any more.

As a doctor, I find alcoholism and co-dependence are a very real challenge. I have found that although these sicknesses are of very long duration — go on for years and years usually — only now and then does a crisis happen which brings the alcoholic to the doctor's attention. His denial keeps him away. This denial is very much a part of an alcoholic's problems, but one reason for writing this book is to appeal to the wives of alcoholics to throw their own denial away, and learn something about alcoholism. If wives stopped being so powerless and learnt about what can be done, then the crises which happen could be turned to good effect. Alcoholism makes the alcoholic behave irrationally: his wife is in a much better position to carry out a plan of improvement. I think we doctors have not supported Al-Anon enough, and until now often not known how to help.

In the next chapter several other ways of helping are described.

Things you can do

1 Fill in the Significant Other Questionnaire given overleaf. What is your 'other's' score?
2 Have you felt powerless, helpless, or hopeless about influencing your husband's drinking?
3 Is the problem serious?
4 Identify your negative coping responses (page 81). Try to substitute positive responses (page 82).
5 Attend Al-Anon. Go to at least a dozen meetings, as it takes at least this long to grasp even the basics of the programme. If you really want to change, do not give up. If you meet any very bitter people in Al-Anon groups, do not let them put you off. Choose the Al-Anon members you

like. The address of Al-Anon is in the telephone book under 'Important Numbers' Personal Emergency Service, or see Appendix 3. Nar-Anon contact address is in the appendix at the back of this book.

6 Consider talking to an alcoholism counsellor about your position. Try the local Alcohol and Drug Centre (see telephone book or Appendix 3, page 134).

Significant other questionnaire

		YES	NO
1	Do you worry about your spouse's drinking?	___	___
2	Have you ever been embarrassed by your spouse's drinking?	___	___
3	Are holidays more of a nightmare than a celebration because of your spouse's drinking behaviour?	___	___
4	Are most of your spouse's friends heavy drinkers?	___	___
5	Does your spouse promise to quit drinking without success?	___	___
6	Does your spouse's drinking make the atmosphere in the home tense and anxious?	___	___
7	Does your spouse deny a drinking problem because he/she drinks only beer?	___	___
8	Do you find it necessary to lie to employer, relatives or friends in order to hide your spouse's drinking?	___	___
9	Has your spouse ever failed to remember what occurred during a drinking period?	___	___
10	Does your spouse avoid conversation pertaining to alcohol or problem drinking?	___	___
11	Does your spouse justify his or her drinking problem?	___	___
12	Does your spouse avoid social situations where alcoholic beverages will *not* be served?	___	___
13	Do you ever feel guilty about your spouse's drinking?	___	___
14	Has your spouse driven a vehicle while under the influence of alcohol?	___	___
15	Are your children afraid of your spouse while he or she is drinking?	___	___
16	Are you afraid of physical or verbal abuse when your spouse is drinking?	___	___

17 Has another person mentioned your spouse's
    unusual drinking behaviour?   ____   ____
18 Do you fear driving with your spouse when he
    or she is drinking?   ____   ____
19 Does your spouse have periods of remorse
    after a drinking occasion and apologise for
    behaviour?   ____   ____
20 Does drinking less alcohol bring about the
    same effects in your spouse as in the past
    required more?   ____   ____

Based on these experiences we suggest the following scale in answering the above twenty questions.

If you have answered YES to any two of the questions, there is a
definite warning that a drinking problem may exist in your family.

If you have answered YES to any four of the questions, the
chances are that a drinking problem does exist in your family.

If you have answered YES to five or more, there is very definitely
a drinking problem in your family.

Key words

Crisis: Serious trouble which is a special point in time for
making a new decision; turning point.

Coping response: What a person does in response to problems
and troubles.

Denial: Act as if spouse's alcohol problem is only a minor
trouble.

Enable: Act to allow drinking to continue; protect alcoholic from
consequences.

Family Members' Programme: The co-dependent goes to hospital instead of the alcoholic. This gives her isolation from him to
rebuild her shattered self-esteem.

Powerless: Feeling you are not in control.

Separation: Wife leaves husband (or vice versa). May be temporary or permanent.

Tough love: Love the alcoholic enough to let him feel the consequences of his addiction. Stopping 'enabling' but continuing to
love your alcoholic.

CHAPTER 13

Co-dependency (2):

Action for recovery by wives of alcoholics

Recovery starts with yourself. You can gain control over your own emotions and behaviour if you follow the Al-Anon programme and the other suggestions given here. But you can *never* control your husband's drinking. Sometimes different choices confront the family members and you are well advised to talk things over with people you trust to be both helpful and confidential before taking hasty action.

> For years I held the family together. I smoothed over the kids' ruffled feelings; I went out to work to pay the bills; I went to the kids' rugby games and the parent/teacher meetings; I made the decisions about holidays. Ken used to come home from the pub at 6.30, have his tea, switch on the TV and drink his half-g then go to sleep, with the TV blaring away. The kids used to laugh at him behind his back. I used to look at him and think of the man I married . . . it was so different then. [Weeps] I seemed paralysed. I could not think of anything I could do. My friends told me to leave him. But I love him, and in any case, where would I go? Besides, he hadn't really done anything, I mean he's never even laid a finger on me. He kept saying he'd cut down, did for a bit, but it always came back again.

What are the options open in such a situation? The first is to learn about alcohol problems, which you have started to do by reading this book! Try Al-Anon books and leaflets also. Contact your nearest Alcohol and Drug Centre (see addresses listed on page 134) and talk about your situation to a counsellor. You will be surprised how sharing your load will help you to carry on, and solutions will appear. To continue the story above:

> I got very depressed and my doctor sent me to the Alcohol and Drug Centre. I met some other ladies who talked to me. What a relief to find I wasn't so alone, so different.
>
> The counsellor taught me about not being a slave to Ken's drinking. Not long after that I stopped waking him up when the TV finished, and getting him off to bed. I just left him there. Sometimes he'd come in to bed at 3 a.m., sometimes he'd sleep there in his clothes. A couple of times he wet himself and the chair. I asked him to come to the Centre with me after that. He agreed to, and came two or three times. Cut his drinking down, and we had some good talks. But he wouldn't stop, not altogether, so I wasn't surprised when he gradually went back. But it didn't worry me so much. The boys and I have a much better life. I don't nag. I know Ken is sick. One day I hope he'll want to do something about it. But I'm not going to be sick with him. I still love him. And he's the boys' father.

Ken's wife no longer feels totally limited by Ken's drinking. She has new hope, a new understanding, and a new communication. She is clear that alcoholism is his sickness, and she can learn to live a reasonably happy life in spite of it. Indeed, somewhat amazingly she may be a better person because of it.

The following shows how a crisis can be used to bring about attitude change:

> After George's fourth DIC [drunk in charge of a motor car] we had a flaming row. We'd had lots before, but this one was —well, something snapped. I waited until he went to work and then I took the children and some belongings to my mother's. I'd just had enough. Of course he came around that night, but Dad talked to him. He said he'd do something about his drinking, really meant it this time. I told Dad I needed some space, and that I'd heard it all before. Dad apparently advised him to come back in a couple of days' time, when we'd both had a chance to cool off. Meantime I rang my friend who has had some of the same problems. She said to use it to get George to see the counsellor, but not to make any promises about going back. So when he came round again, I said we should both go to see the counsellor together. I made an appointment, and we went a couple of

days later. They suggested inpatient treatment for him, and out-patient for me, with couples' groups. We also had a session with our kids. After that I got to believe he was serious about his drinking. So I went back. He doesn't drink at all now, our communication is better — and when he gets his licence back I won't have to worry about him causing accidents any more.

The flow chart opposite shows how various situations and strategies can be used to help. It looks complicated, but it is a step-by-step approach. Start at the beginning and follow it through!

Some of the terms in the flow chart need explaining.

12th Step call

This is an Alcoholics Anonymous concept (see step 12 on page 26). AA members take it in turns to visit people who telephone for help, and talk about how they got their own recovery. For 12th Step calls to be successful the alcoholic needs to be motivated to ask for help himself. From bitter experience, AA members know it is rarely successful if the co-dependent wife asks for her husband to 'be talked to'.

> I went to the address as requested by the Group Secretary. The door was answered by a very tearful lady. 'Have you come from AA?' she asked. When I said I had, she showed me into the lounge. You could just about cut the atmosphere. I could hear this argument in the bedroom — well, it would have been impossible not to actually. She came back very crestfallen and told me her husband wouldn't speak to me. I left a leaflet, and told her she should try Al-Anon herself.

Concerned confrontation

This is a special technique where an alcoholism counsellor, the family member, and some concerned friends of the family meet together without the alcoholic. The counsellor asks each person to produce three facts about the alcoholic's drinking, and also discusses some sort of ultimatum. Once all this is clear, there is a second meeting (often later the same day), to which the alcoholic is invited. One type of ultimatum comes from an employer, who can also be present: 'Either you go for

Flow chart for action by a co-dependent wife

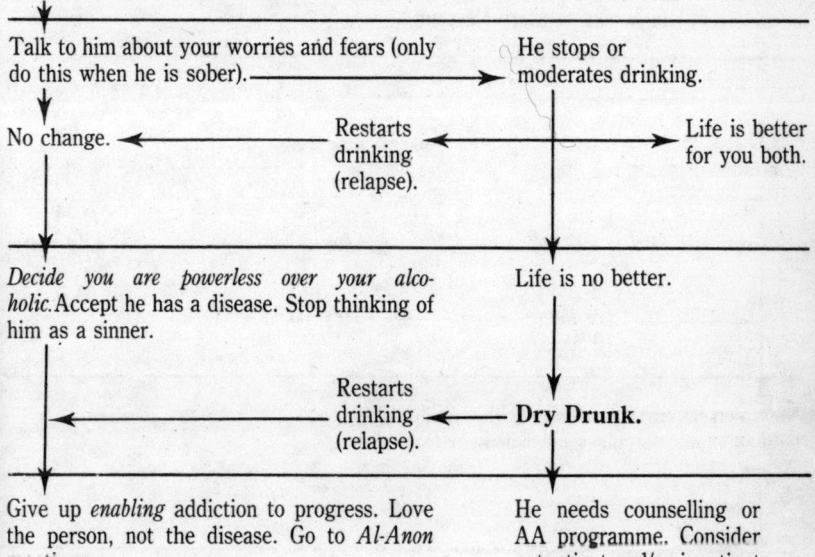

Wife (Co-dependent)   **Husband (Alcoholic)**

Agree you live with a husband who has a drinking problem (see Chapter 1).

Talk to him about your worries and fears (only do this when he is sober). → He stops or moderates drinking.

No change. ← Restarts drinking (relapse). ← Life is better for you both.

Decide you are powerless over your alcoholic. Accept he has a disease. Stop thinking of him as a sinner.   Life is no better.

← Restarts drinking (relapse). ← **Dry Drunk.**

Give up *enabling* addiction to progress. Love the person, not the disease. Go to *Al-Anon* meetings.   He needs counselling or AA programme. Consider outpatient and/or inpatient treatment.

Learn *tough love* — that is, ensure he feels the consequences of his addiction. Stop fixing things up. Learn *loving detachment*. Learn a spiritual position so you and children keep on an even path. Be as happy as you can. Remember unhappy people choose (or cause their own) isolation. Ensure you have supportive relationships. Keep going to Al-Anon. Consider church groups. Consider *personal growth counselling*. See local alcoholism counsellor, if there is one. Become aware of your *negative coping responses*. Substitute positive ones.

Realise it will need a *crisis* before change occurs. You do not need to sink with your husband. Firmness is kinder than permissiveness — set the limits but *do not become his 'mother'* — you are a wife, not a parent!

Get regular support for yourself while this is going on. Either await a çrisis, or consider *concerned confrontation* (*only* with professional help) or arrange own inpatient admission to a *Family Members' Programme* such as that run by Queen Mary Hospital.

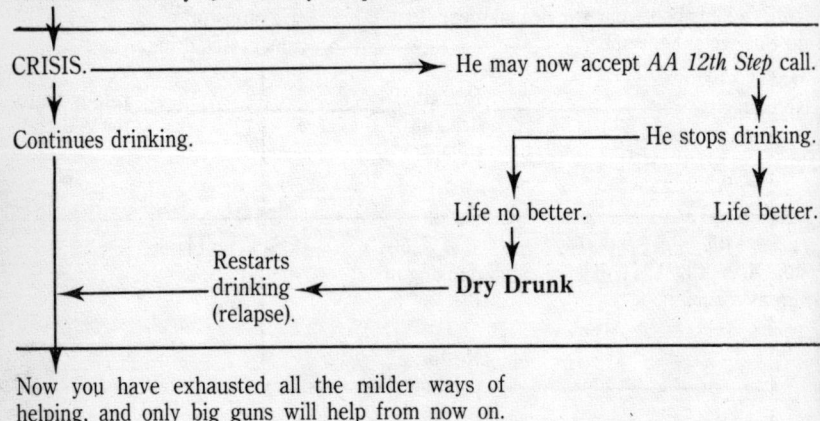

CRISIS. ————————————————————→ He may now accept *AA 12th Step* call.

Continues drinking.   He stops drinking.

Life no better.   Life better.

Restarts drinking (relapse). ←———— **Dry Drunk**

Now you have exhausted all the milder ways of helping, and only big guns will help from now on. Strong alcoholic denial needs strong measures to change it.

Concerned confrontation with *separation* as lever. Remember separation need not be forever; that will depend on his response and your own love. Inpatient treatment is the goal of all concerned confrontation sessions
OR *Alcoholism and Drug Addiction Act* invoked.

He accepts inpatient treatment.

Stops drinking. —→ Life better.

←———— Restarts drinking (relapse). ←————

Be prepared to talk through his resentments about either of these methods. Maintain loving detachment. Remember there is no progress until he takes responsibility for his own disease. Attend Family Therapy at hospital if he goes as inpatient.

Life no better.

Dry Drunk.

If *separation* occurs, remember you are vulnerable to form unhealthy dependency relationships with men. Cultivate women's company, attend Al-Anon regularly, explore grief at ending of marriage, ensure children understand what has happened. See lawyer about rights under Matrimonial Property Act, etc. Consider marriage guidance counselling.

Husband may try self-pity; martyrdom; threats of violence; verbal abuse, or remind you of your marriage vows, to force you back. Keep his drinking and alcoholism in view but his recovery may well be just too late if love has been killed.

Suggest absolute *minimum of two years before any other male relationship* is contemplated. Beware of marrying another alcoholic — hundreds do! Beware of '13th Steppers'.

Your children are at risk of developing alcoholism and drug abuse themselves. Ensure they are educated about this. Try to get them to *Al-Ateen* and occasionally to open Al-Anon meetings. AA/Al-Anon sometimes have social/fun times together — a good learning experience for your children.

Ensure continuing, supportive friendships. Unhappy people choose isolation. Have fun away from dependency relationships. Continue Al-Anon. Consider church groups. Consider personal growth counselling and maintain progress. Realise you are not alone nor isolated and it is possible to be happy without having a partner! Maintain spiritual position.

treatment, or you lose your job.' Another, more common, type of ultimatum comes from a wife who is at the end of her tether: 'Either go for treatment, or we separate.' Naturally this must never be said unless it is going to be carried through. Never make a bogus threat. Children and teenagers can be involved in this concerned confrontation, which must be a loving procedure. The participants must show tough love for their alcoholic. It is the fact that the alcoholic is loved that will get him into treatment. Use of this method should be followed by inpatient treatment: do not allow the alcoholic just to make empty promises. A maximal effort by you and friends should be followed by a massive educational, therapeutic and emotional input — not just a promise not to drink. That will have been given (and broken) many times before. Promises are part of minimising the denial; it is time for the alcoholic to show how serious he is for change. Going into hospital, where his attitude will be constantly monitored, will assist attitude change.

I recommend using concerned confrontation *only* when organised by trained counsellors: it is a powerful technique and, like all powerful things, can go wrong if not sensitively and skilfully handled.

Dry Drunk

When an alcoholic stops drinking, but remains difficult to live with, the term Dry Drunk is often used. When a wife says (or feels like saying) to her sober husband 'You were easier to live with when you were drinking', then he is probably a Dry Drunk. He has stopped using alcohol to help him cope with his feelings and hurts but hasn't yet learned to cope with them by himself, so he is tense, moody, arrogant and so on, and needs treatment and counselling (see Chapter 8).

Alcoholism and Drug Addiction Act

Two doctors and a relative may apply to the District Court for the detention and treatment, at a mental hospital, of an alcoholic whose drinking is causing injury to his health, or is a source of harm, suffering or serious annoyance to others, or makes him incapable of properly managing himself or his affairs. Obviously such a step will produce anger and resentment in the alcoholic, and should never be taken lightly. On the other hand, the Act is certainly under-used in New Zealand. Its use should be discussed with your doctor and alcoholism counsellor. It can be both life-saving and marriage-saving, provided both parties communicate sufficiently.

Separation

Leaving your husband or threatening to leave must be your decision, and yours alone. Certainly discuss it with friends, and your alcoholism counsellor, but only you can decide if love has finally died. Sometimes it is better to have a trial separation, without committing yourself to a permanent separation. The worst use of separation is when it is a type of geographical escape or flight from reality.

When marriages start to go wrong, the mature reaction is to ask, 'What is wrong?' This is best discussed with a counsellor, looking carefully at your own response to the marriage breakdown. Simply blaming your alcoholic partner will not produce any personal growth nor really resolve the situation. In alcoholic marriages, the alcoholic acts immaturely because of his alcoholism *plus* whatever personality difficulties he has. Before separating, a co-dependent wife needs to know about her reaction to these things and to embark on a programme to sort them out. Once she is getting her serenity back, then she can decide if love is dead or not.

You would be surprised and depressed by the number of women who swap one alcoholic husband for another. It is said 'Love is blind', and I suppose this must be the explanation — although I prefer to ask people to distinguish between infatuation and love. Always talk to friends, and introduce any prospective lover to them — then you will see if he fits into your life. Ending a relationship makes a woman very vulnerable. Take time to 'heal' yourself before entering another relationship. A useful guide is to deliberately settle for a two-year gap between commitments. This allows personal growth to take place. Remember the saying that, 'If you love someone, set them free, and if they really love you, they will endure and return.' If you have plenty of friends and a full social life, with support and communication at a platonic level, then you will not need to rush into sexual relationships for the wrong reason.

Relapse

What should you do if your recovering alcoholic relapses? The first thing is to keep serene. Remember that drinking or not drinking is his responsibility — there is no way you can control it. It is important to tell him in an adult, neutral way, that you know he is drinking. You must talk to him about your fears, and also talk to your Al-Anon friends. But I repeat, you cannot control his drinking. Instead you monitor his behaviour. As soon as any alcohol-induced problem occurs, apply tough love, stick with Al-Anon, consider a concerned confrontation, etc. (turn back to flow chart on pages 91–93 for suggestions).

You may await behaviour changes before acting in relation to his drinking. However, your own personal recovery and serenity can be worked on constantly: keep talking to your friends about your inner fears and emotions.

Things you can do

1 Consult the flow chart and see where you are at. What action is recommended?
2 Are you going to take this action? If not, write down the reasons why. Discuss them with a trusted friend.
3 What support systems do you have available to you: Al-Anon, local drug and alcohol clinic, your doctor, your local church and minister?
4 How do you have fun each day?
5 Reread Chapters 7 and 8, much of which applies to family members too, e.g., the differences between admitting and accepting alcoholism, the importance of talking rather than acting out your feelings and so on.

Key words

A & DA Act: Alcoholism and Drug Addiction Act — a New Zealand law which allows two doctors and a relative to apply to a judge to have an alcoholic committed to therapy.

Concerned confrontation: A special interview to force an alcoholic to choose between either taking treatment or else losing his or her job or spouse.

Crisis: Serious trouble which is a special point in time for making a new decision; turning point.

Dry Drunk: Behave as if drunk or hungover, but not having had anything to drink at all. Often shows as a loss of previous serenity, which is replaced by angry mood swings, return of tension and perfectionism, being over-critical of others, being childish and demanding, etc.

Family Members' Programme: The co-dependent goes into hospital instead of the alcoholic. Gives her isolation from him to rebuild her shattered self-esteem.

Separation: Wife leaves husband (or vice versa). May be temporary or permanent.

Tough love: Love the alcoholic enough to let him feel the consequences of his addiction.

12th Step call: A visit from a recovering alcoholic to a drinking one, to try to persuade the drinker to join Alcoholics Anonymous. Because of dangers of being misunderstood, best to be made by men to men, and women to women. This avoids dangers of '13th Steppers'.

13th Stepper: Use of 12th Step call between members of opposite sex which results in sexuality interfering with the AA message.

CHAPTER 14

Co-dependency (3):
For husbands of
alcoholic wives

Husbands feel a great deal of shame when their wives have problems with alcohol. Separations in these marriages occur in a much shorter space of time than in marriages where the man is alcoholic.

Husbands are also much slower to accept help from outside agencies. Perhaps male pride has a lot to do with it, but it is harder for me to get a man to attend Al-Anon, than it is to get a woman alcoholic to attend AA. Men in this position need help to understand that addiction is a disease, and they are powerless over it. Men tend to withdraw from their alcoholic wives, and often overwork. Power struggles develop where getting drunk seems a way of the alcoholic gaining a victory over her self-righteous husband. Because so many marriages are less than equal, with the male dominant, this may be one of the few ways in which the female can 'win'. This process is unconscious, i.e., not as deliberate as it sounds when described this way, and like many unconscious processes, is actually self-destructive in the long run.

> My husband is such a perfectionist. I can't do anything right. If I go out of my way to please him, he says I am doing too much. If I don't, he tells me I'm neglecting him. I've just given up.

In the above example you can no doubt detect the alcoholic's self-pity, rationalisation, and projection of blame onto her husband. A therapist or friend will also be aware of the truth that may lie at the heart of the complaint — but the addict's way of dealing with this is to have another drink (or smoke dope, or take tranquillisers).

Co-dependent husbands need to learn 'tough love' and some of the other techniques described in the previous chapter. They will need joint counselling to unravel communication blocks, need to swallow their pride and go to Al-Anon. They will need to encourage and trust their wives to attend AA alone. They will need to recognise their own loneliness and anger, and be aware of vulnerability in relationships with other women. Having an affair is not therapeutic, any more than changing partners is. You just take your problems into a different bed. Personal growth does not occur in beds either, strangely enough!

The denial shown by women alcoholics can be very severe, and puzzling.

> Jill would refuse to discuss the problem at all. The kids were beginning to play up, so I sent them to boarding school. She made out I was the cruellest husband in the world. When I pointed out why they had to go, she told me I was silly. And drank more, not less. My doctor and I told her we'd put the Alcoholism and Drug Addiction Act on her unless she went for treatment. She could see I was serious, so she went, but she called me all the names under the sun. I went to Family Week, and she agreed she had an alcohol problem (although she never said she was an alcoholic). She came home, but she drank secretly. Finally I confronted her, and faced her with the half bottle of gin I'd found. She told me it was mine, and I'd forgotten I'd bought it. I moved out to my parents' place and told the kids what had happened. I still see Jill every few days, and we get on well —but I can see she is deteriorating. I have started going to Al-Anon and the counsellor at the Alcohol Service is a great help. I hope she comes right. At least we don't play some of the destructive games we used to.

In this case the children were communicated with, and his shift out of the family home ensures that the alcoholic feels the consequences of her drinking. But notice that he hasn't cut his ties, nor has he run off with another female. He is awaiting the outcome of his actions, and still loves his wife. Putting 'tough love' into practice is — tough!

Things you can do

1 As the husband of an alcoholic wife, is your pride keeping you from seeking help?

2 Starting on page 134, you will find a list of Alcohol and Drug Centres. Make an appointment to talk over your situation with a counsellor.

3 Read *Al-Anon faces Alcoholism*, obtainable from Al-Anon, then start putting a plan of action together.

4 Consult the flow chart on pages 91–93. Make allowance for the change of sexes, but decide where your alcoholic has got to. What action is recommended?

CHAPTER 15

Co-dependency (4):

For children who have an alcoholic parent and for adults who grew up in an alcoholic or dysfunctional family

If you are a child, and one or both of your parents are alcoholic, then you will be affected by it. Children learn living mainly from the home, and if it is an alcoholic one, their experience of family life is not the best. The more severe the alcoholism, the more obvious this is. But the early stages of alcoholism (see Chapter 1) also affect family life, and therefore affect the way kids learn to live. For instance, relating to an alcoholic parent can be hard because of their mood swings. Is this going to be one of the times Dad is angry, or sad? Will he fly off the handle over nothing, or will he be embarrassingly guilty and remorseful about his drinking or about 'the night before'? Most alcoholics feel very guilty about what they are doing to their families — but don't talk about it. Will he 'buy' your affection with expensive presents?

The home influence is so powerful that about half the sons of alcoholics become alcoholics themselves. About half the daughters of alcoholics marry alcoholics themselves. This is a terrible self-perpetuating cycle: I hope the efforts at public education by such bodies as the Alcoholic Liquor Advisory Council will help to change this.

Even if kids avoid alcohol and alcoholics, they may react to their upbringing by adopting certain lifestyles. For instance, they may be attracted towards 'lame ducks'; they may feel powerless to influence others; they may have a chip on their shoulder; they may be careless of life and limb; they may be angry fighters on behalf of others (e.g., some may become politicians or union officials with a grudge); or they may be angry fighters on their own account (e.g., a businessman fiercely motivated to succeed). They may also be life-long teetotallers because of what they have seen. Such people are now called 'adult children of alcoholics'.

Adult children of alcoholics

Being raised in a dysfunctional family means learning dysfunctional ways of relating to others. Children learn by unconsciously copying what they see around them. During teenage years they may equally unconsciously rebel against the family rules or the wider system (e.g., school), dimly sensing the dishonesty of the family communication style, or the double standards of ordinary adult life. Adolescence is a difficult enough time for any child, struggling to become independent in a complicated world. When one or both parents are chemically dependent, communication at home between family members is so poor that this is bound to be reflected in the children's development.

> When I was 18 I decided to shut down from all the hurts I had received from my mother. I couldn't take any more. She was alcoholic and my father was a workaholic. We moved around a lot — I think I went to ten different schools. I always felt alone and unwanted. I've poured my love into my own children and my husband. I wanted it to be different for them. But John tells me I am unreachable. I feel numb and hopeless, and, well, just different from other people.

In this example the speaker is a nurse, and a wonderful caregiver. In therapy, she is asked to look after herself, her 'little lonely child within', with some of the love and care she shows to others. She is asked to reflect on her childhood training in an ACOA household. Did she unconsciously learn:

> *Don't trust*
> *Don't talk*
> *Don't feel*

— because it is safer to be this way? Her later shutting off is a self-protection device. Often this means that by the time adult life comes, ACOA people have learned how to please others, how to look after them, and how to take no notice of their own needs. Other people are more important, more talented, and more deserving. ACOA people are often very nice people, but keep in the background, trying to control their circumstances by being responsible for everything. They are afraid to trust life. They may adopt different roles as they grow up, in their quest to fit in.

> I realise now, when I look back at my life as a child, how my mother leant on me. I was like a father to her, and my younger brothers and sisters. I'd make sure they all behaved and didn't upset Dad.

There is an element of being a *peacemaker* here too — a sort of Walt Disney *hero*, always doing what is right. Another role is the *adjuster*. This is someone who changes whatever they are doing or thinking to suit others. This sort of behaviour is often called co-dependency. The person is dependent on someone else to provide meaning in their lives. They often find alcoholics to look after, unconsciously re-creating their childhood circumstances.

Finally there is the *rebel* or *scapegoat*, who attracts all the family anger. Such ACOAs often develop addiction problems of their own later in life, but all ACOAs are vulnerable to developing both addictive and co-dependent traits later in life.

ACOA problems are very common in our society. Self-help groups and therapy groups for ACOAs are available in many centres. Psychotherapy and counselling can also help a person to develop new healthy roles to replace the unhealthy ones. This doesn't happen overnight obviously. It will take months or years to correct faulty patterns learned over many years. The length of therapy will depend on the severity of the problem, and the abilities of both therapist and patient. A typical programme might be as follows. Start with outpatient counselling, taking a detailed history, and appreciating what patterns emerge. Trust then develops between therapist and patient. Continue with weekend therapy groups over several months, attendance at groups for adult children of alcoholics, attendance at Al-Anon, and keeping on with these things for as long as required to change unconscious reactions. A therapist may recommend attending an inpatient programme for family members, like that at Queen Mary Hospital, if progress cannot be maintained (see Chapter 17). Remember that step 10 of the AA programme (see page 25) reminds us we are allowed to make mistakes, and to grow slowly. We don't have to be perfect all at once. (In fact, perfectionism is a good co-dependent trait!)

Young children in alcoholic families

Most young children are scared when they hear their parents having rows. They also feel somehow responsible. This is partly due to the normal way children's minds work. For instance, very small children appear to think that everything that happens near them is related to them. Thus, some children say that the sun follows them wherever they go — they cannot grasp the idea that it is always there for everybody else as well. So if parents are arguing, the child feels he is part of it — and gets upset. If the family does not communicate well, the child does not tell anyone, and so these sad, angry thoughts remain bottled up, ready for the magic release by chemicals in teenage or early adult life. The other way children feel responsible is because an adult makes a hurtful remark that wounds deeply, and is remembered.

> My mother told me that Dad began to drink worse after I was born.
>
> Mum said she'd have left Dad if she hadn't had to look after me.
>
> Dad told me I was useless because I wet the bed. I hated him for teasing me. He told me it was no wonder he had to drink when he had children like me.

Small children in families where there are emotional outbursts have a great burden to overcome. If they are lucky, they learn the art of living normally from school life or visiting friends' families. If they are not so lucky, they become unhappy, lonely adults, who are very vulnerable to alcohol and other mind-changing drugs. Although there may be a small inherited part to alcoholism, the influence of the home and upbringing is more important in its transmission from one generation to the next.

Teenagers in alcoholic families

In families where the parents' communication is affected by alcoholism, older children are at risk in several ways:

- Adolescent rebellion
- Super good kid — the opposite of the above
- Sexual abuse — incest
- Early sexual promiscuity — solo motherhood
- Loneliness and sadness
- Early marriage to escape

Teenage times are normally characterised by mood swings, testing limits, intense feelings of love and anger and the awakening of sexual feelings. It is a time when children need a stable, loving background against which to test their movement towards independence. Instead they may have to direct their energies to propping up a mother who is despairing about her husband's alcoholism. Or to looking after brothers and sisters and household chores if the mother is the alcoholic. When children have to become parents to keep the family going, they miss out these years of development. This sort of teenage training can turn them into caretaking adults who end up finding another 'lame duck' with whom to spend their lives. Often it is as if the only way such people can be comfortable is to re-create their teenage situation.

A common story is for a kid to do well at primary school, less well at intermediate and hopelessly badly at secondary school. Such a change is often because of family strife.

> I got on okay until Dad left when I was 11. He used to beat up my mum, but he never laid a hand on me. I dunno, I just seemed to go to pieces. When I was 14, I started wagging school. Mum used to give me talks. But when she accused me of having sex, and I hadn't, well I went flatting. Me and my girlfriend smoked a lot of dope after that.
>
> I used to look at my dad, sleeping it off in his chair in front of the telly. Occasionally there'd be great rows between him and Mum. He'd hit her, and me. He'd tell me I was a useless no-hoper. I

told myself I'd never be like him when I grew up. But, you know, I smoked a bit of dope, got busted by the police, got into the booze — I mean where can you listen to music except in the pubs these days? — and now I've got a booze problem. I hate myself. I'm no better than my dad.

Clearly something drives a person blindly in the direction of addiction in spite of a wish not to fall into the same trap. It is this 'something' which is the sickness of addiction.

Incest is said to occur in 15 per cent of all families: a frightening fact. It seems common in alcoholic families, especially where a mother is sexually cool to her alcoholic husband, and a teenage daughter is available. Some alcoholic fathers are highly manipulative, and cultivate their daughter's natural affection for them, with gifts and bribes. If Mum walks out, sometimes the worst can happen.

I remember when Mum announced she'd had enough, and was off. The house was very silent. Dad made a joke about it at first. But he came home rotten on Thursday night after I'd gone to bed. He came in and sat on the bed. I was terrified. Then he got into bed with me . . . [weeps] I went flatting after that.

My mum used to have these awful parties. Sailors used to come. Me and my brothers used to barricade ourselves in my bedroom to keep them out.

After Dad was killed, Mum sort of gave up. She sent us to live in a foster home. This man there used to abuse me and my sister. We felt so low and degraded. He said if we ever told anybody, he'd break every bone in our body. So I never have, until now. I can see how it has made me secretive all my life. It's a wonderful relief to talk about it after all these years.

If these sorts of things are happening to you or your friends, do not suffer alone. Find a trusted professional counsellor and talk to him or her. Or use one of the phone-in services that are increasingly available. Make sure you do not try to handle it alone.

Kids from alcoholic families often try to find love through sex.

I met this sheila and we had sex the same night. I moved in the next day. But it didn't last. That's the story of my life.

Or it may seem that life will have meaning if you can give enough love to someone:

> I got pregnant because I wanted something to love of my very own. It was fun and games at first. Then as Damian got older I found I couldn't leave him, and I couldn't afford babysitters, so I got very lonely. That's when I started to smoke dope and get into the booze.

A relationship that is obviously sick to outsiders from the 'normal world' may seem to provide satisfaction through caregiving and martyrdom:

> I met Rob at a school dance. He was real sad and crazy, but sort of fun, you know. He was always getting drunk and doing screwy things. We started living together, I could see he was sick and needed me to look after him. I enjoyed that — being necessary and important, instead of getting shouted at by Mum for not helping at home. But after a while Rob stopped supporting me, I had to pay all the bills, and give him money for booze. He started hurting me during sex and I got scared of him. Scared to leave and scared to stay.

Things you can do

1 Can you communicate with your non-drinking parent?
2 If not, and you want to try to get through, you can go and talk to a counsellor about it. Either a school counsellor or someone at the Family Counselling Centre or Alcohol Counselling Centre. A minister or a doctor or public health nurse may help (if he or she is interested and skilled in this — but many are not, so you will have to ask around about who is good).
3 Ring up Al-Anon Family Groups and ask about Al-Ateen meetings (see 'Important Numbers' in the telephone book). Or write to Al-Anon for information (see address on page 134 of this book).
4 Ring up Youthline (see telephone book, under 'Important Numbers' at the front).
5 Ring up the local Alcohol and Drug Centre about workshops or sessions for Adult Children of Alcoholics. Try to meet other ACOAs and compare experiences. Don't be afraid if you begin to feel overwhelmed: this is you feeling

your feelings again after all these years of numbness or being shut down. Get appropriate support for yourself — don't be alone with your sadness.

6 Learn how to grieve. Doing grief work healthily and fully will help you release from it.

7 Here are some good books to read. These can be borrowed from your local public library — ask the staff there to help you find them.

Our Shout: Women and Alcohol, by Helen Warren, Chris Griffith and Ingrid Huygens (Heinemann Reed).

This book is highly recommended. It is a New Zealand book written for New Zealand women, and follows on from this brief chapter.

Co-dependent No More, by Melody Beattie (Collins Dove, Melbourne, Australia).

It Will Never Happen to Me, by Claudia Black (Ballantine Books, New York, US).

Women Who Love Too Much, by Robin Norwood (Arrow Books).

8 Complete this Children of Alcoholics Screening Test:

		Tick	
		YES	NO
Q 1	Have you ever thought that one of your parents had a drinking problem?	☐	☐
Q 2	Have you ever lost sleep because of a parent's drinking?	☐	☐
Q 3	Did you ever encourage your parent(s) to stop drinking?	☐	☐
Q 4	Did you ever feel alone, scared, nervous, angry or frustrated because a parent was unable to stop drinking?	☐	☐
Q 5	Did you ever argue or fight with a parent when he or she was drinking?	☐	☐
Q 6	Did you ever threaten to run away from home because of a parent's drinking?	☐	☐
Q 7	Has a parent ever yelled at or hit you or other family members while he/she was drinking?	☐	☐

Q 8   Have you ever heard your parents fight
       when one of them was drunk?   ☐   ☐

Q 9   Did you ever protect another family member
       from a parent who was drinking?   ☐   ☐

Q 10 Did you ever feel like emptying or hiding a
       parent's bottle of liquor?   ☐   ☐

Q 11 Do many of your thoughts revolve around a
       problem-drinking parent or difficulties that
       arise because of his or her drinking?   ☐   ☐

Q 12 Did you ever wish that a parent would stop
       drinking?   ☐   ☐

Q 13 Did you ever feel responsible for and guilty
       about a parent's drinking?   ☐   ☐

Q 14 Did you ever feel your parents would get
       divorced because of alcohol misuse?   ☐   ☐

Q 15 Have you ever withdrawn from and avoided
       outside activities and friends because of
       embarrassment and shame over a drinking
       problem?   ☐   ☐

Q 16 Did you ever feel caught in the middle of an
       argument or fight between a problem-
       drinking parent and your other parent?   ☐   ☐

Q 17 Did you ever feel that you made a parent
       drink alcohol?   ☐   ☐

Q 18 Have you ever felt that a problem-drinking
       parent did not really love you?   ☐   ☐

Q 19 Did you ever resent a parent's drinking?   ☐   ☐

Q 20 Have you ever worried about a parent's
       health because of his or her alcohol use?   ☐   ☐

Q 21 Have you ever been blamed for a parent's
       drinking?   ☐   ☐

Q 22 Did you ever think your father was an
       alcoholic?   ☐   ☐

Q 23 Did you ever wish your home could be more
       like the home of friends who did not have a
       parent with a drinking problem?   ☐   ☐

Q 24 Did a parent ever make promises to you
       that he or she did not keep because of
       drinking?   ☐   ☐

Q 25   Did you ever think your mother was an alcoholic? ☐ ☐

Q 26   Did you ever wish that you could talk to someone who could understand and help the alcohol-related problems in your family? ☐ ☐

Q 27   Did you ever fight with your brothers and sisters about a parent's drinking? ☐ ☐

Q 28   Did you ever stay away from home to avoid the drinking parent, or your other parent's reaction to the drinking? ☐ ☐

Q 29   Have you ever felt sick, cried, or had a 'knot in your stomach' after worrying about a parent's drinking? ☐ ☐

Q 30   Did you ever take over any chores and duties at home that were usually done by a parent before he or she developed a drinking problem? ☐ ☐

Score: Six or more YES answers means you are a child of alcoholic parents.

Acknowledgment: The Children of Alcoholics Screening Test (CAST) is printed by kind permission of the author, Dr John W. Jones (copyright 1983) and published by Camelot Unlimited, 5 North Wabash Avenue, Suite 1409 — Department 18RC Chicago, Illinois, USA 60602.

CHAPTER 16

Pills and potions for denying emotions:
Chemical dependency

It seems increasingly easy for young people in our society to get hold of different drugs, particularly cannabis (pot, dope, marijuana). Because it is common, people think it is safe and normal. This chapter tells you some of the things that are not safe or normal. If you want to put these substances into your brain, and break the law by doing so, that is your risk and privilege. But if you behave poorly and live dishonestly as a result, that becomes a problem for the people you live and work with as well. If you have read the earlier chapters you will be on the alert to ask yourself why it is you have found it necessary to smoke dope. Substituting one drug for another, e.g., stop alcohol, start dope, achieves nothing. This is called polydrug use (poly is the Greek word for 'many'). Polydrug use is a trap, because it disguises the fact that different drugs all have the same purpose — to deal with underlying feelings. The different drugs add up in the body, and you may develop chemical dependency before realising it.

Here are some of the reasons people give for polydrug use:

- To feel happy.
- To escape from miserable reality into a temporary oblivion.
- To be one of the crowd — 'everyone else is'.
- To belong to a tight 'family' — the drug world.
- To show society or parents you do not care.

- As part of the adolescent rebellion.
- To seek a personality change, e.g., so you are no longer a shy person.
- To feel grown up.
- To solve your problems.
- To learn more about yourself.

Throughout this book, I have suggested that all such problems are better handled by talking to others, to counsellors, and looking for personal growth by attending suitable therapy. I have not seen anybody who found satisfactory adjustment through drugs or alcohol. Usually if they have found serenity it is in spite of the alcohol and drugs, not because of them!

Cannabis

Pot is definitely addictive, just as alcohol is. Most people smoke only a little, and the risk is small, just as for alcohol. But some people smoke a lot, get a behaviour change, cannot imagine life without it — they are addicted. You can be addicted to pot and switch dependencies to other drugs and vice versa.

> I knew I had a booze problem, so I stopped drinking. But I kept on smoking [pot]. My wife smoked too. I got so tense and one day I hit her. I didn't know what I'd done. It wasn't me. She cleared out because her first husband did that to her.

A young female patient I treated for cannabis dependency told me she got paranoid (fear that other people are talking about you) as a result of smoking. This was so frightening she decided to stop. But she restarted smoking and the paranoia recurred (i.e., it was a drug-induced effect). So she came to hospital. She did not think she had an addictive problem, because she still believed cannabis was not addictive. It took her urine test four weeks to come clear of cannabis, and this had no sooner happened than she went on leave, smoked dope and felt guilty. On return to the hospital she was asked for a urine specimen which revealed her relapse. She was discharged — a consequence of activating her addiction, instead of talking it through with the loving support available. She learned the power of her addiction the hard way. She has since been drug-free.

Cannabis is stored in the fatty parts of the brain and body, and leaks out over four to six weeks. Whereas chronic alcoholics get alcohol out of their system in two to three days, and their brains begin to clear in three to four weeks, the heavy cannabis user still has cannabis detectable for four to six weeks after the last smoke. Clear thinking seems to take several weeks more. This long period as cannabis leaks slowly out of the brain is why withdrawal symptoms are so subtle. It is like an automatic de-tox, where the level in the body is gradually reduced. In an alcoholic, the rapid withdrawal of alcohol may give shakes, vomiting, hangover and occasionally DTs. This doesn't happen with cannabis. As with alcohol, there is the thought or craving for another smoke, but not usually the 'morning after' (although this can happen). It will come the next night, or in a few days' time. If taken, the level of cannabis present in the brain will be topped up.

It has to be six weeks from your last smoke for you to be the owner of a clear brain. My patients confirm this. It takes them all this time to begin to think straight. It is this constant living in a mild fog of cannabis effects which is the biggest problem with cannabis. If the user is a teenager, then he or she will tend to use drug effects to deal with the painful emotions of teenage years. Unfortunately we only become mature adults by facing our emotions. If we run away from them, and hide behind a cloak of cannabis, then we haven't done the necessary work. This is why so many cannabis users are immature and self-centred; they have a 14-year-old mind in a 25-year-old body.

> I started wagging school at 14. We went flatting when I was 17 — couldn't stand Mum's way any longer. I'd have the odd boyfriend. I'd listen to music stoned, I'd feel sorry for myself. Why can't my family be normal? I've just drifted until now; I'm 24 and I'm still expecting to change Mum. I see I've got to get my support elsewhere. I've got quite a few friends who are straight — got more who smoke, though. It is going to be hard, but I want to leave the dope alone now. I want to be myself, not a sort of zombie.

I am quite convinced that brain damage occurs with cannabis: poor concentration, poor problem solving, poor short-term memory and *lowered* threshold to stress (although cannabis may be a tranquilliser to begin with, later on it can promote violence, as in the example on page 112). Heavy users also get a curious lack of motivation to do anything. They drift around without thought for the future, in an ambitionless state, often expecting others to provide and care for them. This gets them further and further from the mainstream of life. Such people depend on the chemicals to give them their buzz for living: whereas only good, satisfying and honest relationships with other human beings will actually do this. Cannabis has a very distorting effect on our perceptions. What a smoker thinks is great at the time may not be so at all, in reality.

> I am a shit-hot trumpet player, Doc. One day I and the group got high before a concert. We played like angels. Some bugger recorded it all, and I remember thinking this would be a fantastic recording. Next day we listened — I've never been so disappointed in all my life.

An American researcher gave cannabis to a series of college men and asked them and their girlfriends about its effect on their sex lives. The women apparently did not smoke. The men thought the cannabis helped their sexual performance. The women said it made it worse. This illustrates the illusion of performance: the chemical has an effect inside the user's head, and nothing to do with reality.

Cannabis intoxication affects the ability to drive a car, and recent research has shown that alcohol plus cannabis has a worse effect than either by themselves. It is certainly my impression that brain damage occurs sooner in people who take both together. Research shows that heavy users of cannabis also tend to use other chemicals, particularly alcohol.

A great many people, perhaps 15 per cent of adults, smoke cannabis in New Zealand, and in doing so break the present laws. Some people want to decriminalise cannabis on the grounds that it is no more harmful than alcohol. But we know alcohol does cause a lot of harm (here is a whole book about it!). I have earlier pointed out that if alcohol were discovered today for the first time, it would be a controlled drug along with other tranquillisers. Why make legal another harmful drug and make it easier for more people to become addicted?

Lastly, medical reports are appearing on the bad effects of cannabis smoke on the lungs. Chronic bronchitis, lung tissue damage and increased incidence of lung cancer have been reported. Even before these serious conditions occur there will be a general reduction in lung efficiency.

> I used to be a good runner, but since I've been on the weed, I can't be bothered. When I do run, my breathing feels a lot less free than it used to. I guess I'm really unfit.

Sleeping pills

Mogadon, Halcion, Tuinal, Seconal, Sodium Amytal, Chloral Hydrate, Triclofos, Noctec, you name it — all are cross-dependent with alcohol. That is, if you are tolerant of large doses of alcohol, you will be tolerant of large doses of sleeping pills. All are addictive. All remain in the body for long periods, e.g., Mogadon for two to four days, depending on your age (shorter for younger and longer for old). Hangover and accumulation therefore occur. I have seen DTs occur in a 70-year-old who was abruptly taken off the two tablets of Mogadon she had been taking daily for a number of years.

Alcohol can induce sleep too, but only for three to four hours. After this the subject tends to awake and need another dose — dependency has occurred. Our society is obsessed with sleep. Unless sleeplessness is a symptom of depression or psychiatric disturbance, it really does not matter too much. Better to be a little tired than drug dependent! Many recovering alcoholics have told me that soon after they have been given sleeping pills, they feel a return of craving for alcohol. If your doctor tries to do this, show him or her this book, and suggest the alternatives — relaxation therapy, a small dose of chlorpromazine (25–50 mg), or that the sleeping disorder is due to clinical depression (see 'Antidepressants' on page 119).

Appetite suppressants

These drugs (Tenuate, Ponderax, etc.) are all stimulants and are absolutely not for alcoholics or drug-dependent people. If you want to lose weight there are no magic solutions. You must use more energy than you eat. Therefore you must feel

hungry. The sellers of pills and diets really make a killing out
of suckers. Cut out the junk food and chocolate, reduce the fat
and calorie intake and feel a little hungry. It is simple — and
hard. Like most things. If you want to stay trim, you must
make changes in attitude to food and lifestyle and exercise.
Some types of eating disorders go together with addiction,
such as anorexia nervosa (dangerous preoccupation with
being overweight although friends say you are thin enough),
and bulimia (eating lots and then vomiting to get rid of it).

> My weight used to go up and down like a yo-yo. I guess I was
> a fat teenager — then I read about dieting. I remember thinking
> I never need be fat again if I dieted properly. I got down to 40
> kg and got hospitalised. After my first love affair I got to 120 kg.
> I used to go on binges — I'd eat six loaves and make myself
> vomit. Sometimes I'd go to three different restaurants in an even-
> ing and eat a big meal in each. Sometimes I'd take trannies and
> sometimes drink a bit. But mostly I abused food. Inside I felt
> dreadful. I knew it was stupid but I couldn't help it.

Appetite suppressant pills would obviously be useless here.
What is required is long-term support and an attitude change
to life. A lowered self-esteem is often at the bottom of it all. I
recommend such folk for group and individual therapy over
several years, mostly as an outpatient, but with some periods
of inpatient therapy.

Tranquillisers and other magic potions

If you are tense, find the cause and see what can be done
about it.

> I am a stock agent and after hours I do a spot of contract paint-
> ing. I am developing our section, and hope to start building next
> year. I don't see the wife all that much, but she's happy knowing
> we are going to get our own home next year. I get a bit tense,
> Doc, and my stomach can't handle the booze like it used to, can
> I have some trannies?

Working too hard will not be helped by pills, and I wonder
if his wife really agrees with the above assessment! All tranquillisers affect alertness and decision-making, whatever the
makers say.

Tranquillisers have their place in psychiatric illness, but

certainly are not cure-alls. They may help symptoms for a short time, but this is a trap for the addict. They lead back to thinking that there is a chemical to fix life's problems, which obviously is not true. Quite a lot of research shows they are addictive, and cause brain damage. Just as sleeping pills can cause craving for alcohol in the alcoholic, so also can tranquillisers, since many of them are from the same chemical family.

My advice is that no recovering alcoholic should ever be given minor tranquillisers. Instead, use alternatives — talking and counselling; personal growth and spiritual concepts; and if drugs are required, then it is best to use small doses of chlorpromazine or allied drugs (Phenothiazines) or antidepressants. There are too many minor tranquillisers to list, but the commoner ones to avoid are: any members of the benzodiazepine group of drugs, i.e., Mogadon, Valium, Librium, Ativan, Serepax, Rohypnol, Halcion, Noctamid, D-pam, Adumbran, etc. Avoid also Hemineurin, Equanil (Meprobamate) and barbiturate drugs except when used to withdraw alcoholics safely from alcohol, preventing DTs and withdrawal symptoms. This is satisfactory for a *few days* but not any longer. We have admitted people who have brought as many as 180 capsules of Hemineurin with them — this means they have now got two problems instead of one — alcohol dependency and Hemineurin dependency.

'Hard' drugs

All the hard-drug users I have known have also used and abused many other drugs, especially alcohol. Because hard drugs are illegal, and addiction causes insatiable demand, there are bound to be periods of shortage of supply. Addicts must substitute another drug — most commonly alcohol — for relief. Hard drugs are very addictive in the physical sense so that intense withdrawals occur quite quickly after starting to inject them. This is what is so awful about hard-drug use: the whole world becomes concentrated on the need for a 'fix'. Nothing else is so important, certainly not relationships nor the amount of effort needed to be happy in the normal world. Who needs that anyway, when you can get it all from an injection?

How simple life would be if we could inject happiness, or

would it be awful if it really was possible? The book *Brave New World* by Aldous Huxley examined this theme. Most people are relieved we have not found the drug with the magic properties listed in his book. Heroin, morphine and methadone certainly are not. Their side-effects are devastating: addiction and withdrawals; poor health; muddled thinking; social isolation and removal from the mainstream of life; promotion of violence and crime.

A counsellor at a drug clinic has this to say about hard-drug users:

> They think eat and sleep drugs. The conversation always gets quickly back to drugs whatever we talk about. They are very socially isolated — they don't seem to move outside the user group. They form relationships together. Even when a druggie has a job, he is always thinking about drugs. For the women, prostitution is the natural way to get money. They can't talk about their feelings in a meaningful way. And they are *so* unreliable — I waste hours of valuable appointment time or get frustrated when several people turn up at once. It is incredibly hard to get a person drug free when they still live with their mates who are using.

Codeine

Codeine is found in cough mixtures and pain-killing tablets, and acts like morphine. It causes constipation and morphine-like withdrawals and is powerfully addictive. Some of my patients have become well known to local pharmacists, who have to try to resist the addict's desire to buy up all the patent cough mixtures.

> I used to have a map of the city with the pharmacies marked on it. I would schedule visits at intervals, and write them on the map, like a master plan. They got to suspect me, but I don't think they realised how many shops I went to in a day.

LSD

LSD is a frightening drug that distorts time and space, often in a very disturbing way. 'Bad trips' occur, when severe terror is felt. From time to time people die because they feel they can, under the influence of the drug, do strange things, like flying. They may prove this by leaping out windows, unless their friends stop them. 'Flashbacks' also occur, weeks or months after the last dose. They are sudden recurrences of the drug's effect: strange and fearsome, they have to be endured. Occasionally LSD makes a person quite crazy and they must go to a mental hospital for many months or years. Fortunately the abuse of this drug appears to be getting less common.

Antidepressants

These drugs may be life saving for a small number of alcoholics who are Dry Drunks due to depression. They are quite safe for the alcoholic in the correct dosage because they are *not* addictive.

Obviously they must be prescribed by a doctor or psychiatrist, after the correct diagnosis has been made. Because many alcoholics are unhappy on account of their alcoholism, antidepressants tend to get over-prescribed in my opinion. If you have alcoholism you need treatment for that, not a prescription for pills! The good news about antidepressants is that they are not addictive, nor cross-dependent with alcohol. Examples are : Amitryptiline, Imipramine (Tofranil), Trimipramine (Surmontil), Dothiepin (Prothiaden), Mianserin (Tolvon).

Nicotine

Nicotine in cigarettes is very addictive, which is why cigarettes are hard to give up. Excessive nicotine causes sleeplessness, however, and nicotine withdrawals are characterised by tension, mood swings and restlessness. As with any addiction, admission and acceptance will occur only if the addict is convinced his condition is serious. A sad example was a friend of mine who had bronchitis for a number of years. I tried to convince him to stop smoking, for his health. He did — the moment his X-ray showed he had lung cancer. He died nine months later. Smoking and alcohol are the two biggest controllable public health hazards of our age.

Caffeine

Caffeine in tea and coffee, and some cold cures, is a stimulant and mildly addictive. In excessive doses (ten or more cups of coffee per day), it can cause sleeplessness, heart palpitations and headaches. If you cannot sleep, do *not* get up and have a coffee or tea — have a milk drink like Milo, which does not have caffeine in it.

Cocaine

Cocaine is currently 'fashionable' because it is supposed to produce a happy high and add to sexual pleasures. It is strongly addictive, and whether it actually does do what it is supposed to is rapidly lost sight of because of the craving for it, and the expectations of the user. It is generally taken as a snuff, and this will eventually rot the inside part of the nose if the user ignores warning pains. Unfortunately cocaine is a local anaesthetic, and so blots out this pain. A person high on cocaine is unpredictable, and may therefore be violent. Cocaine is not commonly available in New Zealand, so I have not met a great many patients who have had much of it.

Glue sniffing

This is the current fashion among kids aged between 10 and 14 years. It is unclear to me why it should be popular, since it causes sickness (nausea) along with a high or doped feeling. I suspect it is a passing phase for most teenagers, but use over months and years will produce brain damage and personality change. 'Normal' children may become moody, secretive, preoccupied with drugs, smoking and alcohol, and there is a falloff in school work and ordinary sporting activity.

Conclusion

It is easy to understand why unhappy teenagers like the feeling of 'powdered happiness' that drugs can give. There is the additional thrill of doing something that parents, teachers and authority figures do not approve of. Most young people use drugs only briefly, discover the pitfalls for themselves, and change their activities to other things. They find happiness through steady relationships of their own, and satisfaction in work of some kind. They take some sort of spiritual position which carries them through difficult periods such as illness, the death of a loved one and material misfortunes.

If somebody fails to make these sorts of adjustments, they may turn to drugs and become addicted. Lack of employment, for instance, may hinder such development. Young people who keep using drugs stay immature, often have excuses for this, and often increasingly use alcohol. A favourite excuse for delaying recovery is to point to the approval New Zealand and Western culture gives to alcohol, and say 'other people use alcohol the way I use drugs, so what is wrong?' The answer is that it depends on the effect of these chemicals on a person's behaviour. If other people, like boyfriends, girlfriends, and families are affected, or the use of drugs leads to offences against the law, then obviously something is wrong. Each reader must make up his or her mind on whether others are being hurt by so-called 'recreational' use of drugs. One danger is that early dependency is a subtle and powerful thing, and my fear is that if it becomes the expected norm to take drugs, then many more people will get caught by addiction.

Questions you can ask yourself

1   Do you use any other drugs apart from alcohol?
      Aspirins or similar
      Nicotine
      Caffeine
      Sleeping pills
      Tranquillisers
      Cannabis
      Others
      Prescribed drugs
2   Do you misuse any of them?
3   If you stop drinking, are you at risk of increasing your use of other mind-changing drugs? If so, which ones?
4   Do you have sleeping difficulties? If so, what causes them: tension, excessive caffeine, clinical depression, faulty learning, pain or something else?
5   Have you decided at any time to reduce your use of drugs and found you have gradually increased again? This is a sign of addiction.

6 Joining the normal world means living honestly, within the law. Will you do this? It means burning all cannabis plants and seeds; saying no to anybody who offers you drugs; deciding to earn an honest living and be poorer if necessary.

7 Do you use rationalisation to avoid facing the truth? (You will have to discuss that with a counsellor or a recovering person, since we are blind to our own rationalisations.)

8 Have you ever exceeded the normal dose of aspirins or disprins? (Tabs 2 every 4–6 hours for relief of fever or headache.) What do you use them for? Is this healthy?

9 Cigarettes are known to cause bronchitis, lung cancer and heart attacks. How is it that 90 per cent of alcoholics smoke, but only 37 per cent of NZ adults smoke? Has this smoking something to do with a need for mind-changing chemicals?

10 How well do you care for your body and brain, or do you just take it for granted?

11 In some of the larger cities, Narcotics Anonymous (NA) has begun. NA functions like AA, but is for people with a primary drug problem. Contact addresses may be found on page 145 of this book.

Key words

Antidepressants: Medically prescribed drug for relief of severe depression. Not addictive or cross-dependent; safe for addicts to use under medical supervision. Dangerous in excess.

Appetite suppressants: Pills peddled by drug companies which claim to help slimming. They are addictive, dangerous and do not work!

Cannabis: Pot, dope, grass, marijuana, hash oil, buddha sticks.

Chlorpromazine: Medically prescribed drug for relief of hallucinations and severe anxiety. Not addictive, and occasionally useful in certain types of severe emotional disorder. Known as a major tranquilliser. Other name is Largactil. Is not cross-dependent with alcohol.

Cross-dependence: Nearly all mind-changing drugs can substitute for each other, meaning that dependence on one will transfer to another very easily.

Depression: Severely unhappy mood which colours the whole of a person's life for weeks or months. Guilty, 'black' thoughts, possibly of suicide. Feeling of doom and that things will never be better. Sleep poorly. May lose appetite.

De-tox: Period of time after stopping taking a drug until the body and brain have recovered their normal state. Maybe several days or weeks, depending on the type of drug and the length of time it has been taken for.

Hard drugs: Heroin, morphine, 'home bake', opium, pethidine, temgesic. Usually given by needle into a vein. Severely addictive and dangerous.

Illusion of performance: Belief by the drinker that he or she is functioning better than normal but the outsider knows this is not so.

Nicotine: Addictive drug in tobacco.

Paranoid: Fearing that other people are talking about you, or plotting against you.

Tranquilliser: Usually called 'minor tranquilliser' to distinguish it from chlorpromazine (see above) — often medically prescribed for anxiety and poor sleeping, but after one or two weeks is rapidly addictive even in normal doses. Popular on the black market. Psychologically cross-dependent with alcohol.

CHAPTER 17

Psychotherapy:

What it is and how
to find it

Psychotherapy involves any attempt to relieve another person's mental distress by mental means. Typically this means talking between at least two people. Group psychotherapy means talking with others, typically a group from eight to twenty. The method is based on the fact that most behaviour is learned from other people. We are taught by our immediate family unit as children, and later we are taught by our friends, our acquaintances and our enemies. We learn through living, in fact. Psychotherapy focuses first on learning what has gone wrong, usually by taking a detailed individual history of the whole of a patient's life, from birth (or even before it, e.g., family history, immigration, circumstances of conception/adoption may be sometimes very important) to the present. A skilled interviewer taking a history may already help us to see what has gone wrong, and develop this knowledge, which is called *insight*. New insights often occur as time goes by. Sometimes these are called 'Aha!' experiences, as in 'Aha! Now I see what is wrong'. Often the patient feels very hopeful and buoyed up by these experiences. This is important in itself because most people seeking psychotherapy have been demoralised and feel hopeless for themselves. Being in therapy often means experiencing powerful emotions, both negative and positive. The working through of the negative, being supported by the therapist's interventions, is the real work of psychotherapy, together with consolidating the positive.

Making connections between what happened in the past and what is happening now helps the addict's self worth improve. The realisation comes with relief that we are the product of our past, and are not to blame.

Blame is not helpful when we want to change. I do not allow patients to wallow in self-blame, which is often no more than looking backwards for self-pity and remorse and staying in the 'victim's position'. Instead we must look forward and be responsible for using our insights to make positive behaviour changes. We must change our old, conditioned responses (see Chapter 4, pages 30–31).

This is possible with the support of a good relationship with a psychotherapist. Some people also achieve this with the self-help groups of Alcoholics Anonymous, Narcotics Anonymous, Al-Anon, Adult Children of Alcoholics, Women for Sobriety, Grow and other groups. If this works for you —great. If not, you need more. A psychotherapist is trained to use the relationship that develops between the patient and themselves, to produce both insight and behaviour change. Approved psychotherapists are bound by a code of ethics that endeavours to avoid any exploitation by the therapist.

The way the patient relates to the therapist, and other members involved in group therapy, mirrors the way the patient behaves to others near to them in life. The therapist uses this to help the patient appreciate what is unhelpful and to develop new ways of relating. The level of success will depend on the bond of trust between them, and the willingness of the patient to see the process through, even if it becomes emotionally painful. Skilful therapists must develop the art of being both supportive and probing, and be sensitive to what is not being said, as much as what is being said. To get value from psychotherapy, patients should be prepared to have many months of sessions. It took years to develop your behaviour, and it can't be unlearned and new behaviour adopted in a few sessions. Other parts of life may have to be altered to maintain the gains made in individual interviews, e.g., a willingness to join groups of other people who are also trying to learn new ways to relate and live. Often the value of therapy is directly proportional to the frequency of corrective emotional experiences a group member has.

Here are two examples of corrective emotional experiences.

All my life I have lived in fear of men, even my husband. Well, particularly him, I suppose. He was, I can see now, just like my dad — male, chauvinist, alcoholic and a sexual abuser. I didn't make any progress until I started talking to my therapist about the sexual abuse I had from my dad as a teenager. My therapist, himself a man, taught me to see how this conditioned me to feel dirty and used.

He encouraged me to do a role play in his office, telling an empty chair, which was my dad, how his coming into my bedroom had terrified me. Later I did a psychodrama with a whole group of people. We re-created that scene, and others, and I felt my new power to make a different ending from the earlier one. I grieved my father's abuse of me, and I could also see through that there were parts of him I really loved, still, in spite of it all.

A middle-aged man, John feels isolated and apart. He is encouraged to talk about his early life. He describes a household where his father is quiet, passive, a peacemaker, and his mother is aggressive and dominant. There is nobody to talk to. He remembers feeling close to his father, who dies before this alliance bears fruit, when the patient is ten. Using this in a psychodrama session, he is invited to talk to this father, without his mother being present. Obviously in life this never happened, but in therapy it is a corrective emotional experience. He does so, and a moving and emotional encounter takes place. Later on the psychotherapist reminds John of the necessity of picking a sponsor within AA who can to some extent fulfil the absent father role, and to value fatherly qualities in other relationships he makes. After a year, he reports that he feels much less isolated, much less tense, and is no longer a dry drunk.

The two examples above use psychodrama. Here is a different example from a patient considering her own case and coming to a new conclusion.

Today I realised the real me has been locked up in my own private fortress for most of my life, with my feelings on the outside so that I could not reach them. I can see why I've not been able to love or really feel anything towards other people except when I am drunk. It's like I can come out of my fortress for a while but when I do I can't feel properly, which is frustrating. Tomorrow when I am in group therapy I shall share this with the others and try to let myself come out in front of them. I am afraid of their reactions, but nevertheless I think this is the right thing to do so that I have to stay outside the fortress and learn to deal with life myself without the aid of drugs.

What courage, and what a good vision this person has for herself. This is the beginning of a new and better journey.

Whole books have been written about psychotherapy. The purpose of this brief chapter is to demystify what psychotherapy is, and encourage you to seek it out if you feel you need it.

How do I find it?

Undoubtedly, the best way is to ask people who have had psychotherapy the name of a good local practitioner and what they charge. Unfortunately, very little psychotherapy is offered free by the health services, and most of it is very brief. Individual psychotherapy away from the health services costs anything between $30 and $100 per hour, depending on the therapist's qualifications and skill (and market and ethical forces). Group therapy is usually cheaper per session.

People you can ask for guidance include your general practitioner, the practice nurse, local clergymen and the Citizens' Advice Bureau (address in phone book). Look in the Yellow Pages under Psychotherapists, or Psychologists. Local psychiatrists can advise, as can the New Zealand Association of Psychotherapists (contact: The Executive Officer, NZAP, 23 Essex Road, Mt Eden, Auckland).

When you select a psychotherapist, ask what they offer, what they charge, and see if you can relate well to them. You must be able to have a good relationship, or it will not work. You are buying a service, so appraise it carefully before you start.

APPENDIX 1

Further reading

Alcoholics Anonymous ('The Big Book'). Available in New Zealand from the General Service Office of Alcoholics Anonymous, PO Box 6458, Wellington, or from your nearest AA group.

Twelve Steps and Twelve Traditions, available as above.

Pass It On. The story of Bill Wilson and how the AA message reached the world. Available as above.

Jean Kinney and Gwen Leaton. *Loosening the Grip: a handbook of alcohol information.* C. V. Mosby Co., Saint Louis, USA.

Abraham J. Twerski. *Caution: Kindness can be dangerous to the alcoholic.* Prentice Hall Inc.

Personal growth and understanding

Muriel James and Dorothy Jongeward. *Born to Win.* Addison-Wesley Publishing Co., USA.

John Powell, *Why am I afraid to tell you who I am?* Argus Communications.

Choosing to Change. Published by Radio New Zealand Continuing Education Unit. Send two blank C60 cassettes to the National Film Library, Private Bag, Courtenay Place, Wellington, plus $2 postage and a self-addressed gummed envelope.

Granger E. Westberg. *Good Grief.* Fortress Press, Philadelphia, USA. (A short paperback which has helped many people.)

Co-dependency — for family members

Al-Anon Faces Alcoholism. Available in New Zealand from

Al-Anon General Service Office, PO Box 40-507, Upper Hutt.
Toby Rice Drews. *Getting Them Sober: a guide for those who
live with an alcoholic.* Haven Books.
Judith Sexias. *Living with a parent who drinks too much.* Green-
willow Books, New York.

Drugs
Capsules and Potions and Drugs for Emotions. Published by
Radio New Zealand Continuing Education Unit. Send two
blank C60 cassettes to the National Film Library, Private
Bag, Courtenay Place, Wellington, plus $2 postage and a self-
addressed gummed envelope.

Maori history and alcohol dependency
Burns, Patricia. *Te Rauparaha: A New Perspective.* A. H. &
A. W. Reed Ltd, 1980.
Cowan, J. *The Maori yesterday and today.* Whitcombe &
Tombs, Auckland.
Durie, M. H. 'Te Taha Hinengaro: An Integrated approach to
Mental Health.' Paper presented to Hui Whakaoranga (Maori
Health Hui), Hoani Waititi Marae, Auckland. March 1984.
Gluckman, L. K. 'Alcohol and the Maori in Historic Perspec-
tive.' *New Zealand Medical Journal.* January 1974, pp. 553–55.
Hiroa, Te Rangi. *The Coming of the Maori.* Whitcombe &
Tombs, Wellington.
Hohepa, P. A. *A Maori Community in Northland.* Reed, Well-
ington.
King, Michael. *Te ao huri huri: The world moves on — aspects
of Maoritanga.* Hicks Smith & Sons Ltd, Wellington.
Orange, Claudia. *The Story of a Treaty.* Allen & Unwin in asso-
ciation with Port Nicholson Press, Wellington.
Rolleston, Sam. 'He Kohikohinga: A Maori Health Knowl-
edge Base.' Research Project for Department of Health, 1988–
89.
Tiaki Hikawera Mitira (Mitchell, J. H.). *Takitimu.* Southern
Reprint.

Psychotherapy
Block, Sidney (ed.). *An Introduction to the Psychotherapies.*
Oxford Medical Publications. (This is intended for people who

want to become psychotherapists — quite heavy going for the average reader.)

Williams, Anthony. *The Passionate Technique.* Tavistock Routledge. (This describes psychodrama, and is written by an Australian psychologist, who is a senior lecturer at La Trobe University, Melbourne.)

APPENDIX 2

Checklist of treatment objectives

The following is designed to help you plan and work on your own difficulties. It is your treatment and your life; be active in pursuing good health. It will not fall off the ceiling into your lap!

Addiction
Do you have an:

Accurate knowledge and information about alcohol misuse and drug misuse? (Chapters 1, 2 and 16).

Acceptance of the illness concept of alcohol problems and drug problems? (Chapter 4).

Understanding of any physical damage to your own body? (Chapter 3).

Understanding of any brain damage (poor memory; poor problem solving; changing moods)? (Chapter 9).

Acceptance of your own alcoholism or drinking problem? (Chapter 4).

Attitude to Steps 1–5 of AA programme which is clear and healthy? (Chapter 6).

Understanding of the reasons and circumstances surrounding your alcohol problem? (Chapter 5).

If you are a woman alcoholic, have you read Chapter 10?

The person (Chapters 6, 7, 8)
Behind the bottle or the pills is the person who has to go on

living, and profit from their experiences. Ask yourself if any of
the following apply to you, and if they do or have done, what
action can you take for the present and the future?

Have you any need for assistance with the following areas of
your life?

Unreasonable feelings of anxiety or tension
Depression
Suicidal ideas
Anger
Resentment
Guilt
Sexuality — lack of knowledge; lack of sensitivity; repeating
    unhappy or short relationships
Ability to make good decisions or not
Self-esteem — too low or too high?
Lack of assertiveness
Psychiatric problems
Impulsiveness or irresponsibility
Manipulation of people
Unresolved grief
Expressing feelings of love
Making conversation with strangers
Shyness
Self-pity
Degree of motivation for recovery (procrastination)
Stickability — how easily do you give up?
Educational achievement — reading and writing skills, qualifi-
    cations
Low tolerance of frustration
Clarity about legal position
Clarity about financial position
Clarity about spiritual position
Self-identity — do you know who you are?
Over-inflated ego?
Loneliness
Aware of own potential strengths/weaknesses (see steps 4 and
    5 of AA programme)
Tendency to hide feelings
Understanding of personal dynamics (e.g., understand the

many factors that contribute to your developing an alcohol problem).

Family and friends — social life (Chapters 12, 13, 14, 15)
Understand and improve relationship with spouse.
Understand and improve relationships with family members.
Understand and improve relationships with friends and the world.
Have a healthy peer group.

Treatment progress
Stay the whole course of therapy.
Show in-depth involvement with progress of group and individual therapy.
Have your family or a significant other involved.
Accept and participate in special groups if referred (i.e., grief, psychodrama, social skills, Maori).
Care for your body — physical exercise, accepting disabilities.

After care
Plan support systems on return home if treated as inpatient — know local AA meetings; know local professional help available; have sponsor/understanding friend.
Continue to take personal inventory (step 10).
Plan leisure time.
Know dangerous trigger situations.
Recognise Build Up to Drink for self (BUD).
Work on steps 6–12.
Obtain employment and make a living honestly.
Review educational achievements.
Continue to look for personal growth.
Take Antabuse if recommended.
Have suitable place to live.
Maintain healthy attitude to drugs — caffeine, nicotine, tranquillisers, medical needs.
Be aware of problems in sobriety ('Dry Drunk').
Know how to arrange re-admission.
Decide whether to keep in touch with therapist after discharge.
Enjoy physical activities.

Useful addresses

General information

This book has repeatedly urged you to talk with other people, if you want recovery. Equally, if you want to stay recovering, you should allow yourself to receive support and not be alone. Alcoholics Anonymous and the Al-Anon family groups are available throughout New Zealand, but their locations sometimes change with time; if you find the address given here is incorrect, try the telephone book under Alcoholics Anonymous, Al-Anon Family Groups, or under 'Important Numbers'. Or write for information to the General Service Office in Wellington. (AA's address is PO Box 6458, Wellington, phone 859-455; Al-Anon's is PO Box 40-507, Upper Hutt.) AA and Al-Anon are self-help organisations that make no charges and have no dues. They are not part of any Health Service or Government system.

Your local Citizens' Advice Bureau can also help. As well as telling you where to find your nearest alcohol/drug services, the Bureau has information on neighbourhood organisations which can help if you are lonely or socially isolated. The address and phone number of the Citizens' Advice Bureau will be found in your local phone book.

What follows is a list of places where you can refer yourself if you wish. It is advisable to telephone for an appointment first, but if you don't trust yourself to stick to an appointment, don't delay — just drop in. You may have to wait a little, but at least you will have made contact.

Most area health board centres are open during normal

office hours, but because this doesn't suit everybody, there are usually evening sessions as well. Don't put it off, or think your problem isn't serious enough!

Useful addresses of helping agencies

(Arranged by locality, from north to south of New Zealand.)

Whangarei
Northland Dependency Services,
Northland Base Hospital, PO Box 743, Whangarei
Phone: 482-079

Auckland
Community Alcohol Services (Auckland Area Health Board),
77 Carrington Road, Point Chevalier, Auckland 2.
Phones: 893-720 ext 608, 860-808, 862-932.
Eden Clinic (Auckland Area Health Board),
13 Gilgit Road, Epsom, Auckland.
Phone: 687-023.
National Society on Alcoholism and Drug Dependence,
8 Hall Avenue, PO Box 22-489, Otahuhu, Auckland.
Phones: 276-7192, 276-7193.
Presbyterian Support Services,
Alcohol and Drug Dependency Services,
408 Mt Eden Road, Mt Eden.
PO Box 67-028, Auckland.
Phone: 686-111.
Salvation Army Bridge Programme,
2 Churton Street, Parnell, Auckland 1.
Phones: 793-754, 793-748.
203 Detox — Walk-in Detox Centre,
Auckland City Mission,
203 Federal Street, Auckland.
Phone: 33-016.
Community Addiction Services,
Waitakere Hospital, 55–75 Lincoln Road, Henderson.
Phone: 837-5800.
Auckland Drug Dependency Clinic,
393 Great North Road, Grey Lynn.
Phone: 765-272.
Lake Shore Clinic,
North Shore Hospital,
Shakespeare Road, Takapuna.
Phone 460-553.

N.S.A.D.,
4/115 Church Street Medical Centre,
PO Box 22-489, Otahuhu.
Phone: 276-7192
Te Ara Hou,
94 Browns Road, Manurewa.
Phone: 267-0543.

Tauranga
National Society on Alcoholism and Drug Dependence,
Churchill Building, 45 Grey Street, PO Box 697, Tauranga.
Phone: 780-418.
Tauranga Hospital Board Alcohol Service,
Tauranga Hospital, Cameron Road, Tauranga.
Phone: 84-199 ext 742.

Hamilton
National Society on Alcoholism and Drug Dependence,
109 Victoria Street (cnr Hood and Victoria Streets), Hamilton.
Phone: 390-389.
Corner House — Community Alcohol Services (Waikato Hospital
Board and Presbyterian Support Services),
19 Raukiwi Road, Hamilton.
Phone: 394-352.

Rotorua
Riverholm Community Alcohol Services Centre,
125 Old Taupo Road, Rotorua.
Phone: 83-598.
Te Utuhuia Manaaki Tanga Trust,
125 Old Taupo Road, Riverholm.
Phone: 482-598.
Family Counsellor Addiction Specialist,
104 Tarawera Road, Lynmore.
Phone: 455-113.

Tokoroa
National Society on Alcoholism and Drug Dependence,
12 Slateford Place, PO Box 188, Tokoroa.
Phone: 64-289.

Taranaki
Addiction Service,
Taranaki Base Hospital, New Plymouth.
Phone: 067-36139.

Stratford
Alcoholism and Drug Dependence Unit,
Miranda Centre, Stratford Hospital, Romeo Street, Stratford.
Phone: 0663-7189.

Napier
Community Health Services,
Napier Hospital.
Phone: 352-119.
Springhill Centre,
42 Morris Street, Napier.
Phone: 835-4496.

Wanganui
Alcohol Assessment Unit (Wanganui Hospital Board),
Heads Road, Wanganui.
Phone: 53-909.

Palmerston North
Alcohol and Drug Centre (Palmerston North Hospital Board),
159 Queen Street, Palmerston North.
Phone: 72-066.

Levin
Alcohol and Drug Centre (Palmerston North Hospital Board),
22 Cambridge Street, Levin.
Phone: 89-655.

Masterton
Totara Trust,
96 Lincoln Road, PO Box 725, Masterton.
Phones: 85-881, 85-490. After hours 85-881.

Wellington
Al-Anon Family Groups
General Service Office — PO Box 40-507, Upper Hutt.
Alcoholics Anonymous,
General Service Office — PO Box 6458, Wellington.
Phone: 859-455.
See list (or your local phone book) for individual groups.
General Service Centre — Phone: 846-499.
National Society on Alcoholism and Drug Dependence,
124 Dixon Street, PO Box 9183, Wellington.
Phone: 851-517.
Alcohol and Drug Centre (Wellington Hospital Board),
265 Adelaide Road, Newtown, Wellington 2.
Phones: 898-340, 898-653.

Salvation Army Bridge Programme,
1 Tasman Street, Wellington.
Phones: 850-395.

Alcohol & Drug Service:
H.R.C.M.H.S.,
PO Box 31-022, Lower Hutt.
Phone: 31-022.
N.S.A.D.,
PO Box 1599/17 MacLean Street, Paraparaumu Beach.
Phone: 82-805.
Te Hau Ora Tinana,
PO Box 9400, Wellington.
Phone 801-5155.
Community Health Service,
Warrimoo Street, Paraparaumu.
Phone 058-86746.

Nelson

Alcoholics Anonymous. See phone book.
Alcohol Counselling Service, Nelson Hospital,
Private Bag, Nelson.
Phone: 88-299.

Blenheim

The Community Addictions Counsellor, Wairau Hospital, Blenheim.
Phone: 84-099 ext 881.

Hanmer Springs

Queen Mary Hospital *does not* offer self-referral: you must be
referred by a doctor or an Alcoholism and Drug Addiction Centre.
There is a waiting list of several weeks.

Christchurch

Alcohol and Drug Centre (Canterbury Hospital Board),
258 Armagh Street, Christchurch.
Phone: 50-983.
Salvation Army Bridge Programme,
35 Collins Street, PO Box 9070, Addington, Christchurch.
Phone: 384-436 (after hours also).
Vincentian Recovery Centre,
573 Madras St, Christchurch.
Phone: 852-662.
Kennedy Clinic — Walk-in Detox Centre (Canterbury Hospital Board),
c/o Sunnyside Hospital, Lincoln Road, Private Bag, Christchurch.
Phone: 385-059.

Mahu Clinic,
Sunnyside Hospital, Private Bag, Christchurch.
Phone: 3385-059.
Night Shelter — Christchurch City Mission,
275 Hereford Street, PO Box 1032, Christchurch.
Phone: 795-950.
Women's Action Group on Alcohol and Drugs,
Cranmer Centre, Room 203, Cnr Montral & Armagh Streets,
Christchurch.
Phone: 660-598.

Ashburton
Mid Canterbury Council on Alcohol & Drugs,
Elizabeth Street, PO Box 596, Ashburton.
Phone: 03-308-1270.

Hokitika and West Coast
The Director,
Rata Clinic,
Seaview Hospital, Private Bag, Hokitika.
Phone: 58-740.
Substance Abuse Westland,
141 Revell Street, Hokitika.
Phone: 57-104.

Timaru
Alcohol and Drug Centre,
56 Woollcombe Street, PO Box 503, Timaru.
Phone: 84-611.

Oamaru
Family Health Counselling Services,
PO Box 94, Oamaru.
Phone: 48-993.

Dunedin
Centre for Alcohol Related Disabilities (Otago Hospital Board),
21 Park Street, Dunedin.
Phones: 772-323, 779-633. After hours: Dunedin Public Hospital,
Accident and Emergency Department — 740-999.
Drug and Alcohol Rehabilitation Trust (DART),
PO Box 5265, Dunedin.
Phone: 556-224.

Balclutha
Alcoholism Counsellor, Balclutha Hospital,
Hospital Road, Balclutha.
Phone: 80-500.

Invercargill
Alcohol Assessment Unit,
Southland Hospital, Kew, Invercargill.
Phone: 81-949. After hours: 74-009.

Alcoholics Anonymous

Alcoholics Anonymous is a voluntary fellowship of recovered and recovering alcoholics providing a full range of support groups. Individual members are on call to help the alcoholic in need. Anyone who wants to stop drinking can join AA. Self-referrals are welcomed and no charge is made. The following list has been obtained from the General Service Organisation of Alcoholics Anonymous who have kindly permitted it to be printed.

New Zealand General Service Office,
PO Box 6458, Wellington, Phone 859-455.
Auckland Service Centre,
PO Box 6821 Wellesley Street, Auckland, Phone 734-294.
Christchurch Service Centre,
PO Box 2062, Christchurch, Phone 790-860.
Wellington Service Centre, PO Box 6538, Wellington,
Phone 846-499.
Dunedin Intergroup, PO Box 6115, Dunedin
Greater Wellington Intergroup, PO Box 45-109, Lower Hutt.
Hawke's Bay Intergroup, PO Box 253, Napier.
Rotorua Intergroup, PO Box 189, Rotorua.
Taranaki Intergroup, PO Box 4238, New Plymouth.
Wellington Service Centre, PO Box 6538, Wellington,
Phone 846-499.
Dunedin Intergroup, PO Box 6115, Dunedin.
Southland Intergroup, PO Box 16, Invercargill.

AA Groups meet regularly in the following towns:

City or town	Number of groups	Meeting day	PO Box (if available)
Alexandra	1	Wednesday	
Amberley	1	Friday	
Arrowtown	1		Box 92
Ashburton	5	Monday, Wednesday, Friday	Box 172
Auckland	86	Daily	Contact Service Centre (Phone 734-294)
Balclutha	1	Monday	Box 49
Blenheim	7	Monday, Tuesday, Wednesday, Thursday, Sunday	
Cambridge	1	Sunday	Box 384
Christchurch	46	Daily	Contact Service Centre (Phone 790-860)
Coromandel	2	Wednesday, Friday	
Cromwell	2	Thursday, Saturday	
Dargaville	1	Thursday	
Dunedin	7	Monday, Wednesday, Thursday, Friday, Sunday	Box 1071 Box 2029
Featherston	1	Friday	
Feilding	2	Wednesday, Friday	Box 372
Gisborne	3	Monday, Wednesday, Friday	
Gore	2	Wednesday, Sunday	Box 81
Greenmeadows	1	Monday	Box 255
Greymouth	2	Wednesday, Friday	
Hamilton	5	Monday, Tuesday, Thursday, Friday	Box 834

Hastings	5	Tuesday, Wednesday, Friday, Saturday, Sunday	Box 813
Hanmer Springs	2	Wednesday, Sunday	PO Box 67
Hawera	1	Tuesday	Box 301
Hokitika	2	Wednesday, Thursday	
Inglewood	1	Tuesday	
Invercargill	10	Daily	Box 16
Kaikohe	1	Wednesday	Box 567
Kaikoura	2	Thursday, Saturday	Box 56
Kaitaia	2	Tuesday, Wednesday	Box 553
Kaka Point	1	Friday	c/o Post Office
Katikati	2	Monday, Friday	
Kawerau	2	Tuesday, Thursday	
Kerikeri	1	Tuesday	
Kurow	1	Thursday	Box 838
Leeston	1	Wednesday	
Levin	2	Monday, Friday	
Mahia	1	Sunday	
Mangakino	1	Tuesday	
Mangawhai	1	Thursday	c/o Waipu PO
Marton	1	Monday	Box 53
Masterton	1	Friday	
Matata	1	Saturday	Box 431
Mataura	1	Thursday	
Morrinsville	1	Tuesday	
Mosgiel	1	Wednesday	
Motueka	3	Wednesday, Friday, Saturday	Box 235
Mt Maunganui	1	Tuesday	Box 4278
Murchison	1	Thursday	
Napier	3	Thursday, Friday, Sunday	Box 255
Nelson	3	Tuesday, Wednesday, Thursday	
New Plymouth	2	Monday	Box 4185
		Thursday	Box 191

Ngaruawahia	1	Sunday	Box 54
Ngongotaha	1	Monday	Box 217
Nightcaps	1		
Oamaru	1	Tuesday	
Okaihau	1	Monday	
Opotiki	1	Monday	Box 75
Otaki	1	Thursday	
Otautau	1	Tuesday	
Paeroa	1	Wednesday	
Paihia	1	Friday	
Palmerston North	5	Tuesday, Thursday Friday, Sunday	Box 7025
Panguru	1	Thursday	
Picton	1	Tuesday	
Queenstown	3	Tuesday, Friday	Box 228
Raglan	1	Friday	
Ranfurly	1	Friday	
Rangiora	2	Monday, Wednesday	
Reporoa	1	Friday	c/o Post Office
Richmond	1	Monday	
Riverton	1	Tuesday	
Rotorua	6	Tuesday, Wednesday, Thursday, Friday, Saturday, Sunday	Box 189
Ruawai	1	Tuesday	
Runanga	1	Monday	
Russell	2	Wednesday, Sunday	
Sheffield	1	Wednesday	Box 15
Stratford	1	Monday	
Tahunanui	2	Tuesday, Sunday	
Takaka	1	Thursday	
Taumarunui	2	Monday, Saturday	
Tauranga	2	Wednesday, Friday	Box 139
Taupo	2	Monday, Thursday	Box 565
Te Anau	2	Tuesday, Friday	Box 99
Te Aroha	2	Monday, Friday	
Te Awamutu	1	Thursday	Box 194
Te Kuiti	1	Wednesday	
Temuka	1	Sunday	Box 118

Te Puke	1	Monday	Box 229
Thames	4	Monday, Tuesday, Thursday, Friday	Box 494
Timaru	3	Tuesday, Thursday, Saturday	Box 154
Tokoroa	3	Monday, Thursday, Sunday	Box 603
Turangi	1	Thursday	Box 175
Twizel	1	Tuesday	Box 19
Waihi	1	Friday	
Waimate	1	Wednesday	
Waipu	1	Tuesday	c/o Post Office
Waipukurau	1	Wednesday	
Waikanae	2	Monday, Friday	Box 18
Waiouru	1	Wednesday	Box 26
Wairoa	1	Friday	
Waitara	1	Friday	
Wanganui	5	Tuesday, Wednesday, Thursday, Saturday, Sunday	Box 4
Warkworth	1	Thursday	
Waverley	1	Monday	
Wellington	47	Daily	Box 6538
Westport	1	Monday	
Whakatane	2	Wednesday, Friday	
Whangamata	1	Wednesday	
Whangarei	8	Monday, Tuesday, Wednesday, Thursday, Friday, Sunday	Box 471
Whataroa	1	Wednesday	
Whitianga	1	Tuesday	
Winton	1	Thursday	

Al-Anon and Alateen

Al-Anon is a voluntary fellowship of persons whose lives are being affected by another person's compulsive drinking, usually in the same family. Groups meet regularly to improve the relationship within families, to rebuild self-confidence, to learn about alcoholism and to encourage the alcoholic to seek help. Alateen is a similar group for children who have an alcoholic parent. No charges are made and membership continues for as long as necessary.

There are currently about 130 groups throughout the country. Anyone requiring to make contact with Al-Anon in their own locality should write to either of the addresses given below and they will be put in touch with the appropriate group, or look in the local telephone book.

Al-Anon Information Service,
PO Box 39-373, Auckland West.
New Zealand Al-Anon General Service Office,
PO Box 40-507, Upper Hutt.

Narcotics Anonymous (NA)

General Service Office
PO Box 6826, Wellesley Street, Auckland.
Northern Area
PO Box 47087, Ponsonby, Auckland 1.
Phone: 303-1449.
Central Area
PO Box 133, Palmerston North.
Southern Area
PO Box 26002, North Avon, Christchurch.

A list of meetings can be obtained by writing or phoning either the General Service Office or Regional Offices as above. Meetings are currently available as follows:

Northern:

Auckland	18 per week	Taupo	2 per week
Edgecumbe	1 per week	Tauranga	1 per week
Gisborne	1 per week	Tokoroa	1 per week
Hamilton	1 per week	Thames	1 per week
Rawene	1 per week	Whangarei	1 per week
Rotorua	4 per week		

Central:

Hastings	2 per week	Palmerston North	5 per week
Levin	1 per week	Wanganui	2 per week
Napier	3 per week	Wellington	7 per week.
New Plymouth	3 per week		

Southern:

Ashburton	2 per week	Kaiapoi	1 per week
Christchurch	7 per week	Motueka	1 per week
Greymouth	1 per week	Nelson	4 per week
Hanmer Springs	2 per week	Oamaru	1 per week
Hokitika	2 per week	Timaru	2 per week
Invercargill	2 per week		

NA is expanding in New Zealand.

Overeaters Anonymous

Auckland Intergroup, PO Box 39-380, Auckland, phone 798-931.
NB: Many of the principles of addiction apply equally well to overeating.

Women For Sobriety

This is a new self-help group for women, based around women's issues. Contacts are as follows at the time of going to press:

Auckland
Carrington Hospital
Phone: 860-808.

Eden Clinic
Phone: 687-023

Hamilton
Phone: 394-352 (2 groups)

Rotorua
Phone: 83-598 (2 groups) or 455-133

Taupo
Phone: 82-783

Kaitaia
Phone: 1670

Whitianga
Phone: 65-598 (2 groups)

Rawene
Phone: 819

Nelson
Phone: 880-299 (Alcohol Clinic)

Takaka
Contact Nelson

Christchurch
Phone: 850-983 (2 groups) or
385-059 or 650-983

Invercargill
Phone 81-949 or 82-710

Oamaru
Phone 48-993

Napier
Springhill Clinic

Thames
Phone: 65-598

Free literature and programme guides can be obtained from PO Box 6399, Dunedin. Phone: (024) 737-896